OXFORD MEDICAL PUBLICATIONS

BIOCHEMISTRY OF EXERCISE
AND TRAINING

BIOCHEMISTRY
OF
EXERCISE AND TRAINING

RON MAUGHAN
University of Aberdeen

MICHAEL GLEESON
University of Birmingham

AND

PAUL L. GREENHAFF
University of Nottingham

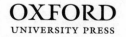

OXFORD
UNIVERSITY PRESS

OXFORD
UNIVERSITY PRESS

Great Clarendon Street, Oxford OX2 6DP

Oxford University Press is a department of the University of Oxford.
It furthers the University's objective of excellence in research, scholarship,
and education by publishing worldwide in

Oxford New York

Athens Auckland Bangkok Bogotá Buenos Aires Calcutta
Cape Town Chennai Dar es Salaam Delhi Florence Hong Kong Istanbul
Karachi Kuala Lumpur Madrid Melbourne Mexico City Mumbai
Nairobi Paris São Paulo Singapore Taipei Tokyo Toronto Warsaw

with associated companies in Berlin Ibadan

Published in the United States
by Oxford University Press Inc., New York

First published 1997
Reprinted 1998

Library of Congress Cataloging in Publication Data
Maughan, Ron J., 1951–
Biochemistry of exercise and training / Ron J. Maughan, Michael
Gleeson, and Paul L. Greenhaff.
Includes bibliographical references and index.
1. Exercise—Physiological aspects.   2. Sports—Physiological
aspects.   3. Biochemistry.   4. Metabolism,   I. Gleeson, Michael,
1948—   .   II. Greenhaff, Paul L.
QP301.M1138   1997   612'.004—dc21   97–31837
ISBN 0 19 262742 2 (hbk.)
ISBN 0 19 262741 4 (pbk.)

Printed in Great Britain
on acid-free paper by
Biddles Ltd, Guildford, Surrey

Preface

This small book aims to provide an introduction to the biochemistry of exercise for students of biochemistry, physiology, and sports/exercise science. It is aimed at the student who has some broad understanding of human metabolism and the physiology of exercise, and who wishes to explore the subject in more depth. There are many texts on the physiology of exercise, but few cover the biochemistry in any detail. Our experience of teaching, however, suggests that students often find it more difficult to come to terms with the biochemistry than with the physiology. There are many reasons for this, but it is undoubted that at an elementary level there are fewer conceptual difficulties in human physiology. The molecular basis of most physiological mechanisms is, however, complex and poorly understood. What is clear is that the laws of chemistry, as they apply to biological systems, ultimately govern all physiological systems.

Our strategy in writing this book has been to take an approach based on physiological chemistry rather than on traditional biochemistry. We are concerned with the reactions and processes that apply to living tissues, and recognize, for example, the differences that exist between different tissues. Our aim in writing this book was to provide a readable text, uncluttered by too much detail. Above all else, we have been concerned to present a broad perspective to allow the whole picture to be seen. The more interested or more advanced student will have to seek detail in specific areas elsewhere, and references to further sources are provided. Some Appendices and a *Glossary of terms* are added to help with specific areas and to provide clarification of some of the less familiar biochemical terminology.

In writing this book, we have also been conscious that rapid advances are being made in the field of physiological chemistry as it applies to exercise, and some of the beliefs we hold to be true today might be shown to be false tomorrow. If the fundamentals—which are likely to remain largely unchanged—are well understood, then new information can easily be fitted into the existing framework, and will help to clarify rather than confuse.

Writing this book has required some hard work, but it has also provided us with enjoyment. We hope that the reader will share with us our enthusiasm and interest.

March 1997	R.M.
Aberdeen	M.G.
Birmingham	P.L.G.
Nottingham	

Acknowledgements

Each author wishes to thank, sincerely, past and present colleagues, mentors, and research students for their positive contribution in making research life, to date, an enjoyable and stimulating experience. Hopefully, their enthusiasm and insight will be reflected throughout the whole of this book.

Paul also thanks Jill for always being there when it mattered and for understanding, on too many occasions, the excessive and unreasonable working hours of academia and research. Lastly, he thanks Sarah for giving so much joy and laughter.

Michael thanks Laura for love and understanding and putting up with all the times he cannot be with her. He also thanks his parents for their unswerving support and Shaun for bringing the joy of parenthood to his life.

The authors also wish to thank Maggie Brown, Adrianne Hardman, and Ed Winter for their comments on early drafts of this book.

Contents

Abbreviations

A	adenine
ACh	acetylcholine
ACP	acyl carrier protein
ADP	adenosine diphosphate
AMP	adenosine monophosphate
	($3'$, $5'$ cAMP, cyclic AMP: an important intracellular messenger in the action of hormones)
ATP	adenosine triphosphate: a high-energy compound that is the immediate source for muscular contraction and other energy-requiring processes in the cell
ATPase	adenosine triphosphatase: an enzyme that breaks down ATP to ADP and inorganic phosphate, releasing energy that can be used to fuel biological work
BCAA	branched-chain amino acid (includes leucine, isoleucine, and valine)
BP	blood pressure
C	cytosine
CCK	cholecystokinin
CGRP	calcitonin gene-related peptide
CHO	carbohydrate
CK	creatine kinase: an enzyme that catalyses the transfer of phosphate from phosphocreatine to ADP to form ATP
CNS	central nervous system (brain and spinal cord)
C_aO_2	content of oxygen in arterial blood
C_vO_2	content of oxygen in venous blood (a bar over the v signifies mixed venous blood)
CO_2	carbon dioxide
CoA	coenzyme A which acts as a carrier for acyl groups (A stands for acetylation)
CoA-SH	free form of coenzyme A
COOH	carboxyl group

CoQ   coenzyme Q or ubiquinone, an electron carrier which mediates the transfer of electrons from flavoprotein to cytochrome *c* in the electron transport chain

Cr   creatine

dm   dry matter

DNA   deoxyribonucleic acid

DOPA   dihydroxyphenylalanine

1,3-DPG   1,3-diphosphoglycerate

2,3-DPG   2,3-diphosphoglycerate

ECF   extracellular fluid

ETC   electron transport chain

FAD   flavin–adenine dinucleotide (oxidized form)

$FADH_2$ flavin–adenine dinucleotide (reduced form)

FDP   fructose 1,6-diphosphate

FDPase   fructose 1,6-diphosphatase

FFA   free fatty acid

FMN   flavin mononucleotide (oxidized form)

$FMNH_2$ flavin mononucleotide (reduced form)

F6P   fructose 6-phosphate

G   guanine

GABA   gamma-aminobutyric acid

GDP   guanosine diphosphate

GLUT 4   glucose transporter found in cell membranes, including sarcolemma of muscle fibres

G1-P   glucose 1-phosphate

G6-P   glucose 6-phosphate

GTP   guanosine triphosphate

H^+ hydrogen ion or proton

HCO_3^- bicarbonate: the principal extracellular buffer

HDL   high-density lipoproteins

HK   hexokinase: an enzyme that catalyses the phosphorylation of glucose

Hz	unit of frequency: cycles per second
HSL	hormone-sensitive lipase
5-HT	5-hydroxytryptamine or serotonin
IDL	intermediate-density lipoproteins
IGF	insulin-like growth factor
IMP	inosine monophosphate
J	joule: unit of energy
kJ	kilojoule: unit of energy ($kJ = 10^3$ J)
K_m	Michaelis constant: the substrate concentration at which the velocity of an enzymatic reaction is half maximal
LCAT	lecithin–cholesterol acyltransferase
LDH	lactate dehydrogenase: an enzyme that catalyses the reversible reduction of pyruvate to lactate
LDL	low-density lipoproteins
LPL	lipoprotein lipase: an enzyme that catalyses the breakdown of triacylglycerols in plasma lipoproteins
M	molar: unit of concentration (nM: nanomolar = 10^{-9} M; μM: micromolar = 10^{-6} M; mM: millimolar = 10^{-3} M)
min	minute: unit of time
mole	amount of substance represented by the molecular mass in grams
ms	millisecond: unit of time
NAD^+	nicotinamide–adenine dinucleotide (oxidized form)
NADH	nicotinamide–adenine dinucleotide (reduced form)
$NADP^+$	nicotinamide–adenine dinucleotide phosphate (oxidized form)
NADPH	nicotinamide–adenine dinucleotide phosphate (reduced form)
NH_2	amino group
NH_3	ammonia
NH_4^+	ammonium ion
O_2	oxygen molecule
OH	hydroxyl group

Pa   pascal: unit of pressure
            (One atmosphere = 101 kPa = 760 mmHg)

PCr   phosphocreatine or creatine phosphate

PDH   pyruvate dehydrogenase: the enzyme complex catalysing the con-
            version of pyruvate to acetyl-CoA

PEP   phosphoenolpyruvate

PFK   phosphofructokinase: the rate-limiting enzyme in glycolysis

pH   a measure of acidity/alkalinity. $pH = -\log_{10}[H^+]$

P_i inorganic phosphate

pCO_2 partial pressure of carbon dioxide

pO_2 partial pressure of oxygen

$\dot{Q}$ blood flow rate or cardiac output

R (group)   organic side chain of an amino acid

RER   respiratory exchange ratio

RNA   ribonucleic acid
            (mRNA: messenger RNA; tRNA: transfer RNA)

RQ   respiratory quotient

s   second: a unit of time

SDH   succinate dehydrogenase: an enzyme of the tricarboxylic acid
            cycle

SR   sarcoplasmic reticulum

T   thymine

TAG   triacylglycerol

TCA   tricarboxylic acid

U   uracil
            (also international unit of enzyme activity: $1\ U = 1\ \mu mol\ min^{-1}$)

UDP   uridine diphosphate

UTP   uridine triphosphate

VIP   vasoactive intestinal peptide

VLDL   very low-density lipoproteins

Vmax   maximal velocity of an enzymatic reaction when substrate concentration is not limiting

$\dot{V}CO_2$ rate of carbon dioxide production

$\dot{V}O_2$ rate of oxygen uptake

$\dot{V}O_2max$ maximal oxygen uptake

Biochemical terminology

Acid	A substance which tends to lose a proton (hydrogen ion)
Aerobic	Occurring in the presence of free oxygen
Allosteric enzyme	An enzyme which alters its three-dimensional conformation as a result of the binding of a smaller molecule (at a site different to its active site), often leading to inhibition or activation of its activity
Anaerobic	Occurring in the absence of free oxygen
Anaplerotic reaction	A reaction that maintains the intracellular concentration of crucial intermediates that might otherwise become depleted (e.g. the formation of oxaloacetate from pyruvate by pyruvate carboxylase)
Base	A substance which tends to donate an electron pair or co-ordinate an electron
Buffer	A substance which, in solution, prevents rapid changes in hydrogen ion concentration (pH)
Carboxylation	A reaction involving the addition of CO_2, catalysed by an enzyme using biotin as its prosthetic group
Catecholamines	Biologically active hormones and neurotransmitters that are synthesized from the amino acid tyrosine. Examples include adrenaline, dopamine, and noradrenaline
cis-	A prefix indicating the geometrical isomer in which the two like-groups are on the same side of a double bond with restricted rotation
Coenzyme	Small molecules which are essential in stoichiometric amounts for the activity of some enzymes
Condensation	A reaction involving the union of two or more molecules with the elimination of a simpler group such as H_2O
Conformation	The shape of molecules determined by rotation about single bonds, especially in polypeptide chains about carbon–carbon links
Covalent bond	A chemical bond in which two or more atoms are held together by the interaction of their outer electrons

Covalent regulation	Control of enzyme activity by covalent bonding of phosphate groups to sites other than the active site of the enzyme
Deamination	A reaction involving the loss of an amino (NH_2) group
Decarboxylation	A reaction involving the loss of a CO_2 group
Dehydration	A reaction involving the loss of a water molecule
Enzyme	A protein with specific catalytic activity. They are designated by the suffix '-ase', frequently attached to the type of reaction catalysed. Virtually all metabolic reactions in the body are dependent on and controlled by enzymes
Epimerization	A type of asymmetric transformation in organic molecules
Flux	The rate of flow through a metabolic pathway
Geometrical isomerism	A form of stereoisomerism in which the difference arises because of hindered rotation about a double bond. An unsaturated fatty acid containing one carbon double bond has two isomers, depending on whether the hydrogen atoms are on the same (*cis*) or the opposite (*trans*) sides of the molecule
Gluconeogenesis	The synthesis of glucose from non-carbohydrate precursors such as glycerol, ketoacids, or amino acids
Glycogenolysis	The breakdown of glycogen into glucose 1-phosphate by the action of phosphorylase
Glycolysis	The sequence of reactions which converts glucose (or glucose 1-phosphate) to pyruvate
Glycosidic bond	A chemical bond in which the oxygen atom is the common link between a carbon of one sugar molecule and the carbon of another. Glycogen, the glucose polymer, is a branched-chain polysaccharide consisting of glucose molecules linked by glycosidic bonds
Half-life	The time in which half the quantity or concentration of a substance is eliminated or removed
Hydration	A reaction involving the incorporation of a molecule of water into a compound

Hydrogen bond	A weak intermolecular or intramolecular attraction resulting from the interaction of a hydrogen atom and an electronegative atom possessing a lone pair of electrons (e.g. oxygen or nitrogen). Hydrogen bonding is important in DNA, RNA, and is responsible for much of the tertiary structure of proteins
Hydrolysis	A reaction in which an organic compound is split by interaction with water into simpler compounds
Hydroxylation	A reaction involving the addition of a hydroxyl (OH) group to a molecule
Ion	Any atom or molecule which has an electrical charge due to loss or gain of valency (outer shell) electrons
Ionic bond	A bond in which valence electrons are either lost or gained, and atoms which are oppositely charged are held together by electrostatic (coulombic forces)
Isoform	Chemically distinct forms of an enzyme with identical activities (also called isoenzyme), usually coded for by different genes
Isomer	One of two or more substances that have an identical molecular composition and relative molecular mass but a different structure due to a different arrangement of atoms within the molecule
Isotope	One of a set of chemically identical species of atom which have the same atomic number but different mass numbers (e.g. 12-, 13-, and 14-isotopes of carbon whose atomic number is 12)
Ketogenesis	The synthesis of ketones
Kinase	An enzyme that regulates a phosphorylation–dephosphorylation reaction
Lipolysis	The breakdown of triacylglycerols into fatty acids and glycerol
Metabolite	A product of a metabolic reaction
Oxidation	A reaction involving the loss of electrons from an atom. It is always accompanied by a reduction. For example, pyruvate is reduced by NADH to form lactate. In the reverse reaction, lactate is oxidized by NAD^+ when pyruvate is re-formed

Peptide bond	The bond formed by the condensation of the amino group and the carboxyl group of a pair of amino acids. Peptides are constructed from a linear array of amino acids joined together by a series of peptide bonds
Phosphagen	The term given to both high-energy phosphate compounds, adenosine triphosphate, and phosphocreatine
Phosphorylation	A reaction that involves the addition of a phosphate (PO_3^{2-} group to a molecule. Many enzymes are activated by the covalent bonding of a phosphate group. The oxidative phosphorylation of ADP forms ATP
Prosthetic group	A coenzyme that is tightly bound to an enzyme
Rate-limiting enzyme	An enzyme in a metabolic pathway that regulates the slowest step in the pathway, and hence limits the rate of flux through the pathway
Reduction	A reaction in which a molecule gains electrons
Stereoisomerism	The existence of different substances whose molecules possess an identical connectivity but different arrangements of their atoms in space
Substrate	The reactant molecule in a reaction catalysed by an enzyme
Thioester bond	A bond in which the oxygen has been replaced by sulfur. For example, the linking of CoA in acetyl-CoA is through a thioester bond.
trans-	A prefix indicating the geometrical isomer in which like-groups are on opposite sides of a double bond with restricted rotation
Transamination	Reaction involving the transfer of an amino (NH_2) group from an amino acid to a ketoacid
Transcription	The process by which RNA polymerase produces single-stranded RNA complementary to one strand of the DNA
Translation	The process by which ribosomes and tRNA decipher the genetic code in mRNA in order to synthesize a specific polypeptide or protein

1
Physiology and biochemistry of skeletal muscle and exercise

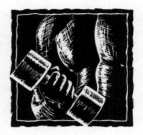

1.1 The physiology and biochemistry of exercise

The disciplines of physiology and biochemistry are virtually inseparable in the field of exercise and sports science. Answers to questions in exercise and sports physiology, including the most fundamental ones, such as the causes of fatigue, can only be obtained by combining the application of these two disciplines. Indeed, one might go so far as to say that the future of exercise and sports physiology resides mostly in the development of our understanding of cellular, subcellular, and molecular mechanisms to explain how the body responds and adapts to acute and chronic exercise. Biochemistry usually refers to the study of events at the subcellular and molecular level, and this is where the emphasis is placed in this book. In particular, we are concerned to explain how exercise modifies metabolism in the muscle fibre. However, muscle also relies on extracellular supplies of fuel and of oxygen delivered by the circulation, so a meaningful description of muscle metabolism must also take into account factors that influence or limit the blood-borne supply of fuel and oxygen. Training modifies metabolic responses to exercise, and training-induced adaptations encompass both biochemical responses (e.g. changes in enzyme activities and the capacity to oxidize lipid) and physiological responses (e.g. changes in maximal cardiac output and maximal oxygen uptake, $\dot{V}O_2$max). Where possible, we have pointed out the links between physiology and biochemistry in the body's response to exercise, and this chapter aims to present to the reader the essentials of anatomy and physiology needed to develop an understanding of the complexity and implications of changes occurring at the subcellular and molecular level.

1.2 Skeletal muscle

Muscle is one of the four primary tissue types in the body—the others being nervous, connective, and epithelial tissue. There are three forms of muscle in the body: cardiac muscle, found only in the heart; smooth muscle, located in the walls of blood vessels, airways, the gut, and the bladder; and skeletal (or striated) muscle, whose fibres link parts of the skeleton. Only skeletal muscle is under direct voluntary control, allowing movement of the limbs to take place as well as maintaining posture. Irrespective of the type of exercise involved, the function of muscle is to exert force and the energy required is provided chemically.

1.2.1 Structure, innervation, and blood supply

Skeletal muscles are separated from their surroundings by a membranous layer of connective tissue, the perimysium or, as it is sometimes known, the fascia. Connective tissue also extends into the interior belly of the muscle as septa of

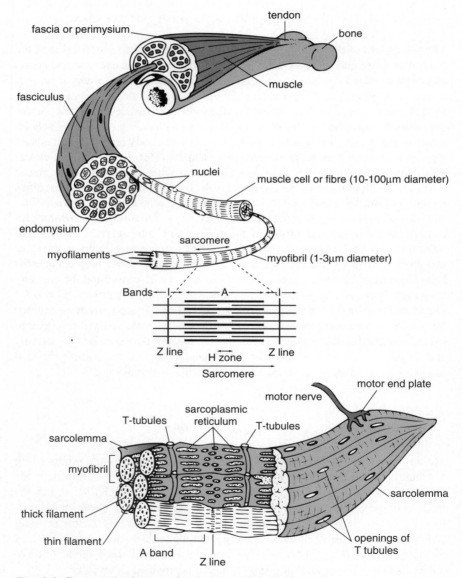

Fig. 1.1 Gross and microscopic anatomy of skeletal muscle.

decreasing thickness (endomysium) subdividing muscle into smaller and smaller compartments (Fig. 1.1). The smallest of these is the fasciculus, each containing a number of muscle fibres bound together and to the endomysium by looser connective tissue. At both ends of the muscle this connective tissue skeleton converges to form tendons.

Tendons are tough bands of tightly packed collagenous fibres which form the connections between muscles and bones. The outer collagenous membrane of living bone (the periosteum) is continuous with the tendinous fibres.

Individual muscles are made up of many parallel muscle fibres that can (but don't necessarily) extend the entire length of the muscle. Inside muscle, the connective tissue also envelops the larger blood vessels and nerves which supply muscle. Almost all muscle fibres are innervated by only one nerve ending located near the middle of the muscle fibre. The specialized synapse separating the nerve and muscle cell membranes is called the motor endplate, and the neurotransmitter released from the nerve ending that initiates force production is acetylcholine. The blood vessels are generally orientated in parallel with the muscle fibres, and numerous capillaries run in the spaces between the individual muscle fibres. The vasculature of muscle constricts or dilates under nervous, hormonal, and local control to regulate blood flow. During exercise blood flow through muscle can increase up to 100 times the resting rate.

Muscle cells are long multinucleated fibres (Fig. 1.1). They vary in length from a few millimetres to over 30 cm and are thin (10–100 μm) cylindrical structures. Each muscle fibre is surrounded by a homogenous membrane, the sarcolemma, which contains collagen fibres in its outer layer that connect it with the intramuscular connective tissue elements. The inner layer of the sarcolemma is the cell membrane proper, across which fuels and waste products are moved and along which the production and conduction of electrical excitation to the muscle fibre occurs. Invaginations of the sarcolemma called the T-tubules allow transmission of the action potential to the interior of the muscle fibre.

1.2.2 Muscle fibre ultrastructure

The interior of the muscle fibre is filled with sarcoplasm (muscle-cell cytoplasm), a red viscous fluid containing nuclei, mitochondria, myoglobin, and about 500 threadlike 1–3 μm thick myofibrils continuous from end to end in the muscle fibre (Fig. 1.1). The red colour is due to the presence of myoglobin, an intracellular respiratory pigment which stores oxygen. Surrounding the myofibrils is an elaborate form of smooth endoplasmic reticulum called the sarcoplasmic reticulum (SR) which is involved in the growth, repair, and replacement of muscle. The SR's interconnecting membranous tubules lie in the narrow spaces between the myofibrils, surrounding and running parallel to them. Under the light microscope muscle fibres have a striated appearance. The striations are due to the unique crossbanding arrangement of the myofibrils. Dark A bands alternate with light I bands along the length of each myofibril; these are the force developing elements. As illustrated in Fig. 1.1, each A band is interrupted at its midsection by a lighter stripe called the H zone, which is only visible in relaxed muscle fibres. The H zone itself is bisected by a dark line called the M line. The I bands also have a midline interruption: a dark area called the Z line. A sarcomere is defined as the region between two successive Z lines in a myofibril, and is the smallest functional unit or segment of a muscle fibre. Each myofibril is effectively a chain of sarcomeres laid end to end. At the molecular level, it can be seen that the banding pattern of the myofibril arises from the orderly arrangement of two types of protein filaments (myofilaments) within the sarcomeres. The thin filaments comprise the proteins actin, tropomyosin, and troponin and extend across the I band and part way into the A band; the thick filaments contain the protein myosin and extend the entire length of the A band. The Z line is a protein sheet in the shape of a disc, it serves as the point of attachment of the thin filaments and also connects each myofibril to the next throughout the width of the muscle fibre. The H zone is the region in which the thick filaments are not overlapped by the thinner ones and is thus lighter when viewed microscopically than the rest of the A band. The M line in the centre of the H zone is evident as a slightly darker line because of the presence of fine strands that link adjacent thick filaments together. Serial cross-sectional views of a myofibril reveal that, in areas where thick and thin filaments overlap, each thick filament is surrounded by a hexagonal arrangement of six thin filaments, and each thin filament lies within a triangle of three thick filaments (Fig. 1.2).

When calcium and adenosine triphosphate (ATP) are present in sufficient quantities, the filaments interact to form actomyosin and shorten by sliding over

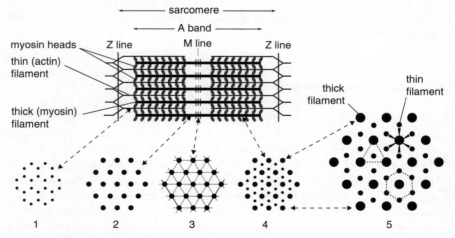

Fig. 1.2 Cross-sectional view of the arrangement of the thick and thin filaments along the length of the sarcomere.

each other. Electrical excitation, passing as an action potential along the sarcolemma and down the T tubules, leads to calcium release from the sarcoplasmic reticulum into the sarcoplasm and the subsequent activation and contraction of the filament array. Excitation is initiated by the arrival of a nerve impulse at the muscle membrane via the motor endplate.

1.2.3 Molecular composition of the myofilaments

Each thick filament contains about 200 myosin molecules, each of which has a rod-like tail, with two globular heads at each end which have ATPase enzyme activity. The myosin heads interact with specific sites on the thin filaments to

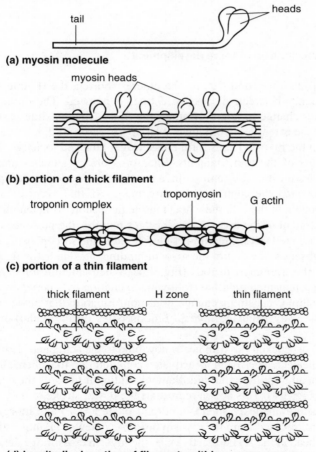

(a) myosin molecule

(b) portion of a thick filament

(c) portion of a thin filament

(d) longitudinal section of filaments within one sarcomere

Fig. 1.3 Molecular structure of thick and thin filaments.

form the so-called crossbridges and generate the tension associated with muscle contraction. The myosin molecules in each thick filament are bundled together such that their tails form the central portion of the filament and their heads face outwards and in opposite directions to each other (Fig. 1.3). Thus, each thick filament has a relatively smooth central section and its two ends are studded with a staggered array of myosin heads. The thin filaments are composed of actin and several regulatory proteins. Globular (G) actin monomers are polymerized into long stands called fibrous (F) actin. Two F actin strands twisted together form the backbone of each thin filament. Successive rod-shaped tropomyosin molecules spiral about the F actin chains and help to stiffen the filament. The other main protein present in the thin filaments is troponin, which contains three subunits. One of these, troponin I, binds to actin, another, troponin T binds to tropomyosin, and the other, troponin C can bind calcium ions (Fig. 1.3).

1.2.4 The mechanism of force development

When a muscle fibre contracts, its sarcomeres shorten, the H zone disappears and the distance between successive Z lines is reduced. The filaments themselves do not change in length. Rather, the thin filaments slide past the thick ones so that the extent of myofilament overlap increases. Sliding of the filaments begins when the myosin heads form crossbridges attached to active sites on the actin subunits of the thin filaments. Each crossbridge attaches and detaches several times during shortening, in a ratchet-like action, pulling the thin filaments towards the centre of the sarcomere. As this event occurs in sarcomeres throughout the cell, the whole muscle fibre shortens in length.

The attachment of the myosin crossbridges requires the presence of calcium ions. In the relaxed state, calcium is sequestered in the sarcoplasmic reticulum, and in the absence of calcium the myosin binding sites on actin are physically blocked by the tropomyosin rods (Fig. 1.4). When calcium ions are released from the sarcoplasmic reticulum (following excitation by a nerve impulse) they bind to troponin C causing a change in its conformation that physically moves tropomyosin away from the myosin binding sites on the underlying F actin chain.

Activated or 'cocked' myosin heads now bind to the actin, and as this happens the myosin head changes from its activated configuration to its bent shape which causes the head to pull on the thin filament, sliding it towards the centre of the sarcomere (Fig. 1.4). This action represents the power stroke of the crossbridge cycle, and simultaneously adenosine diphosphate (ADP) and inorganic phosphate (P_i) are released from the myosin head. As a new ATP molecule binds to the myosin head at the ATPase active site, the myosin crossbridge detaches from the actin. Hydrolysis of the ATP to ADP and P_i by the ATPase provides the energy required to return the myosin to its activated 'cocked' state, empowering

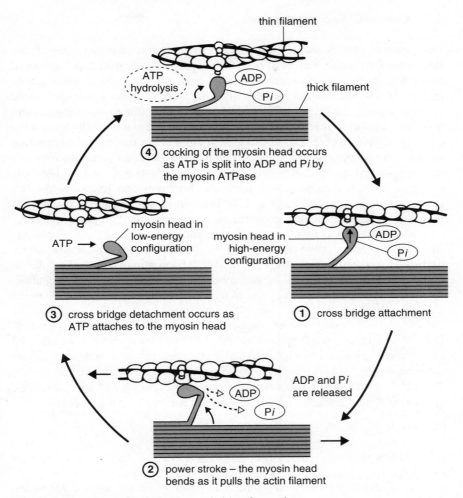

Fig. 1.4 Sequence of events in crossbridge formation.

it with the potential energy needed for the next crossbridge attachment–power stroke sequence. While the myosin is in the activated state, the ADP and P_i remain attached to the myosin head. Now the myosin head can attach to another actin unit further along the thin filament, and the cycle of attachment, power stroke, detachment, and activation of myosin is repeated. Sliding of the filaments in this manner continues as long as calcium is present (at a concentration in excess of 10 μmol^{-1}) in the sarcoplasm. Removal and sequestration of the calcium by the ATP-dependent calcium pump (ATPase) of the sarcoplasmic reticulum restores the tropomyosin inhibition of crossbridge formation and the muscle fibre relaxes.

1.2.5 Control of force development

For a muscle fibre to exert force, a nerve impulse from the motor nerve that innervates the muscle fibre must result in the propagation of an action potential along the sarcolemma. An action potential arriving at the motor endplate causes release of the neurotransmitter acetylcholine which traverses the specialized synapse between the nerve ending and the muscle fibre (the neuromuscular junction) and attaches to acetylcholine receptors on the sarcolemma. This causes the opening of sodium channels, resulting in sodium influx down its concentration gradient into the muscle fibre, depolarization of the membrane, and hence the initiation of an action potential which is then conducted along the muscle fibre sarcolemma in both directions and down the T tubules and results in the full activation of the muscle fibre (Fig. 1.5). Transmission of the action potential to the sites where the T tubules adjoin the sarcoplasmic reticulum causes the latter to release calcium (calcium ion channels temporarily open) and the sarcoplasmic free-calcium concentration rises to above 10 μmol^{-1} allowing crossbridge formation to be initiated as described previously. The continuously active calcium pump returns the calcium to the sarcoplasmic reticulum (usually within about 30 milliseconds), and the inhibition of tropomyosin is re-established when the calcium concentration in the sarcoplasm becomes too low. This sequence of events is repeated when another motor nerve impulse arrives at the motor endplate. When the impulse frequency is high, calcium ions continue to be released from the sarcoplasmic reticulum and the calcium concentration in the sarcoplasm surrounding the myofilaments increases greatly. In this situation, the muscle fibres do not completely relax between successive stimuli and tension will be stronger and more sustained (up to a point) until nervous stimulation ceases.

1.2.6 Motor units

Groups of muscle fibres (of the same fibre type) within the muscle are united through their connection with the same motor neurone. Each group is called a motor unit. Motor units vary in the number of individual fibres from which they are made up: some contain as few as 50 fibres, others up to 1700 fibres. Muscles which perform finely graduated movements (e.g. of the eyes and hands) tend to have small motor units; those involved in coarser movements of larger masses (e.g. the legs) have larger motor units.

An impulse travelling down the motor nerve axon causes depolarization under its motor endplates. All the muscle fibres in the unit will either: (a) not respond, or (b) respond with a conducted action potential along the muscle fibres, followed by simultaneous activation of all the fibres.

A muscle fibre responds to a single stimulus (of sufficient intensity) with a twitch contraction (and relaxation) which lasts about 30 milliseconds. Repeated suprathreshold stimuli cause summation if close enough together, and stimuli at

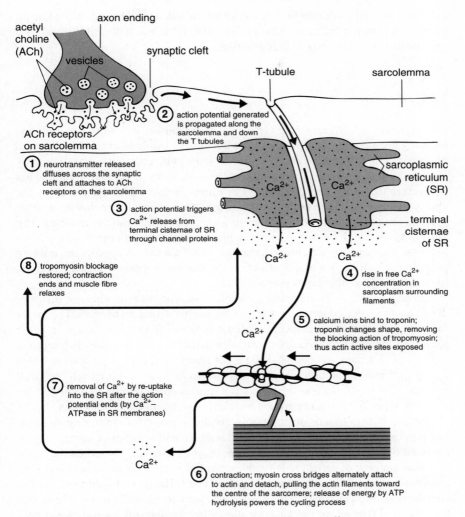

Fig. 1.5 Sequence of events in excitation–contraction coupling.

frequencies of more than 60 per second (i.e. 60 Hz) produce a fusion of twitches (tetanus) with a higher tension than a single twitch.

The normal frequency of stimulation varies from about 5 Hz, which produces low forces, up to about 70 Hz in the production of high forces. An increase in the tension generated by a whole muscle contraction can be effected by: (a) increasing the frequency of stimulation of active motor units, and (b) recruiting an increasing number of motor units.

During exercise of fixed intensity some motor units drop out when fatigued, but their contribution to force generation will be replaced immediately by another until all motor units have been recruited. During maximal-intensity exercise, the initial full recruitment of (almost) all motor units is followed by a gradual loss of some units as fatigue ensues.

1.2.7 Fibre types

The existence of different fibre types in skeletal muscle is readily apparent and has long been recognized, although the detailed physiological and biochemical bases for these differences and their functional significance have, however, only more recently been established. Much of the impetus for these investigations has come from the realization that success in athletic events which require either the ability to generate a high power output or great endurance is dependent, in large part, on the proportions of the different fibre types present in the muscles. The muscle fibres are, however, extremely plastic, and although the fibre type distribution is genetically determined, and not easily altered, an appropriate training programme will have a major effect on the metabolic potential of the muscle, irrespective of the fibre types present.

The original basis for classifying muscle fibre types as red, white, or intermediate was that applied to whole muscles by simple visual inspection. The major functional characteristic that differentiates between fibre types, however, is the speed of shortening and relaxation. Slow-twitch fibres take a relatively long time to reach peak tension (about 80–100 ms for fibres from human muscle) and also a long half-relaxation time. In contrast, human fast-twitch fibres achieve peak tension in about 40 ms and the relaxation time is correspondingly shorter. The two fibre types form distinct groups with little overlap in these properties.

Because of the obvious difficulties in obtaining tissue for measuring mechanical properties, and the relative ease with which small samples of muscle can be obtained by needle biopsy, fibre type classification is usually based on the histochemical staining of serial cross-sections. On this basis, human muscle fibres are commonly divided into three major kinds: Type I, IIa, and IIb (although further subdivisions are possible). These are analogous to animal muscle fibres that have been classified on the basis of their directly determined functional properties as slow twitch, fast twitch-fatigue resistant, and fast twitch-fatiguable fibres, respectively. The myosin of the different fibre types exists in different molecular forms (isoforms), and the myofibrillar ATPase activity of the different fibre types displays different pH sensitivity. The myosin ATPase of the Type II fibres is inactivated at low pH (less than about pH 4.5), whereas the ATPase activity of Type I fibres is unaffected. Above about pH 9 the situation is reversed, and Type II myosin ATPase activity is stable, while Type I myosin ATPase activity is inactivated. By pre-incubation at different pH values close to the lower end of this range, two distinct subtypes of the Type II fibres can be distinguished: the myosin ATPase of the Type IIa fibres is inactivated at pH 4.6–4.8, whereas that of the Type IIb fibres is maintained. It is sometimes possible to detect a Type IIc fibre type by differential pre-incubation, although these do not normally account for more than 1% of the total fibre number in human muscle. It is becoming increasingly common to use gel electrophoresis to distinguish between different fibre types based on the presence of different myosin isoforms. The physiological and biochemical characteristics of the three major fibre types are summarized in Tables 1.1*a* and 1.1*b*.

Type I fibres are red cells that contain relatively slow-acting myosin ATPases and hence contract slowly. The red colour is due to the presence of myoglobin,

Table 1.1a   Characteristics of human muscle fibre types

Characteristic	Type I	Type IIa	Type IIb
	Slow, red, oxidative, fatigue resistant	Fast, red, oxidative, glycolytic, fatigue resistant	Fast, white, glycolytic, fatiguable
Motor neurone size	Small	Large	Large
Recruitment frequency	Low	Medium	High
Contraction speed	Slow	Fast	Fast
Relaxation speed	Slow	Fast	Fast
Maximum power output	Low	High	High
Endurance	High	Medium	Low
Capillary density	High	Medium	Low
Mitochondrial density	High	Medium	Low
Metabolic character	Oxidative	Intermediate	Glycolytic
Myoglobin content	High	Medium	Low
Glycolytic enzyme activity	Low	High	High
Oxidative enzyme activity	High	High	Low
Glycogen content	Low	High	High
Triglyceride content	High	Medium	Low
Phosphocreatine content	Low	High	High
Myosin ATPase activity	Low	High	High
ATPase activity at pH 10.3	0	High	High
ATPase activity at pH 10.3 with pre-exposure to pH 4.6	0	0	High

Table 1.1b   Activities of some glycolytic and oxidative enzymes in different fibre types in human skeletal muscle (μmoles min^{-1} g wet weight^{-1})[a]

Enzyme	Type I	Type IIa	Type IIb
Phosphorylase	2.8	5.8	8.8
Phosphofructokinase	7.5	13.7	17.5
Succinate dehydrogenase	7.1	4.8	2.5
Citrate synthase	10.8	8.6	6.5

[a] Note that the unit of enzyme activity U = μmole of substrate used (or product formed) per minute.

an intracellular respiratory pigment capable of binding oxygen and only releasing it at very low partial pressures (as found in the proximity of the mitochondria). Type I fibres have numerous mitochondria, mostly located close to the periphery of the fibre, near to the blood capillaries which provide a rich supply of oxygen and nutrients. These fibres possess a high capacity for oxidative metabolism, they resist fatigue and are specialized for the performance of repeated strong actions over prolonged periods.

In comparison, Type IIb fibres are much paler because they contain little myoglobin; they tend to be larger in diameter than Type I fibres, although any such differences in fibre size are dependent, to a large extent, on patterns of habitual activity. They possess rapidly acting myosin ATPases, so their contraction (and relaxation) time is relatively fast and consequently they have about a three-fold greater maximum power output than the Type I fibres. They have few mitochondria, a poorer capillary supply, but greater glycogen and phosphocreatine stores compared with the Type I fibres. A high activity of glycogenolytic and glycolytic enzymes endows Type IIb fibres with a high capacity for rapid (but relatively short-lived) ATP production when energy has to be released at rates in excess of that available from oxidative phosphorylation. In other words, they possess a high anaerobic capacity. It is perhaps worth noting here that anaerobic respiration (glycogenolysis and glycolysis) occurs without the use of oxygen, but not necessarily in the absence of oxygen (anoxia), nor for that matter low oxygen availability (hypoxia). Type IIb fibres are best suited for delivering rapid, forceful actions for brief periods, but they are known to fatigue rapidly (see Chapter 6).

Type IIa fibres are red cells whose metabolic and physiological characteristics lie between the extreme properties of the other two fibre types. They contain fast-acting myosin ATPase like the Type IIb fibres, but have an oxidative capacity more akin to that of the Type I fibres.

Recent studies indicate that most muscle fibres actually express more than one myosin isoform. This co-expression of different myosin isoforms effectively gives rise to a wide range of contractile characteristics within a given fibre type (classified according to histological staining techniques) and some degree of overlap between the fibre types in terms of their contractile characteristics. In reality, we are probably dealing with a continuum of contractile and biochemical characteristics, with the two extremes being the classically defined Type I and Type IIb fibres.

Associated with the differences in shortening speed and in the metabolic profile of the major fibre types are differences in the motor neurones which innervate the fibres: Type I fibres are supplied by small diameter neurones which have a slow conduction velocity and a low threshold of activation, whereas Type II fibres are innervated by large diameter, fast conducting neurones that have a relatively high activation threshold. The differences in activation threshold of the motor neurones supplying the different fibre types determine the order in which fibres are recruited during exercise, and this, in turn, determines the meta-

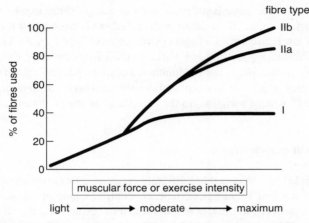

Fig. 1.6 The ramp-like recruitment of Type I (slow-twitch) and Type II (fast-twitch) muscle fibres during exercise of increasing intensity. Note that during the highest intensities of exercise, all fibre types are recruited.

bolic response to exercise. During most forms of movement, there appears to be an orderly hierarchy of motor unit recruitment based on size, which roughly corresponds with a progression from Type I to Type IIa to Type IIb. It follows that during light exercise mostly Type I fibres will be recruited, during moderate exercise both Type I and Type IIa, and during more severe exercise all fibre types will contribute to force production (Fig. 1.6).

Whole muscles in the body contain a mixture of these three different fibre types, although the proportions in which they are found differ substantially between different muscles and can also differ between different individuals. For example, muscles involved in maintaining posture (e.g. the soleus in the leg) have a high proportion (usually > 70%) of Type I fibres, which is in keeping with their function in maintaining prolonged but relatively low forces. Fast Type II fibres, however, predominate in muscles where rapid movements are required (e.g. in the muscles of the hand and the eye). Other muscles, such as the quadriceps group in the leg contain a variety of fibre types. The fibre type composition in such muscles is a genetically determined attribute, which does not appear to be pliable to a significant degree by training. Hence, athletic capabilities are inborn to a large extent (assuming the genetic potential of the individual is realized through appropriate nutrition and training). The vastus lateralis muscle of successful marathon runners has been shown to have a high percentage (about 80%) of Type I fibres, while that of élite sprinters contains a higher percentage (about 60%) of the Type II fast-twitch fibres (see Komi and Karlsson 1978). Such studies, of course, have used the needle-biopsy technique to sample muscle; this method usually provides less than 1000 fibres per sample. A relatively small number of studies looking at the fibre type distribution in whole human muscle have been performed at autopsy. Regional variations in fibre composition appear to be small, although there is a tendency for the deeper parts of the muscle to contain a higher proportion of Type I fibres. This suggests that the needle-biopsy method is a valid method for estimating the fibre composition of a muscle. Studies of the human vastus lateralis indicate that sampling at different sites within the same muscles appears to give no more than about a 6% error (coefficient of variation) in the percentage of the predominant fibre type.

1.2.8 Types of muscle action

Skeletal muscle can perform three different types of action: isometric, where the muscle–tendon length remains constant; concentric, where the muscle shortens; and eccentric, where the muscle is lengthened in the active state. By tradition, muscles are said to contract when they exert force. However, it has been clearly demonstrated that no change in muscle volume accompanies force production in an isolated muscle. During force development, muscle attempts to shorten (i.e. reduce the length of the sarcomeres) and there are basically three possible outcomes. If the attempt is successful concentric activity occurs, mechanical work is done by the muscle, and power is generated. If the attempt is unsuccessful, either the muscle will remain the same length—termed isometric activity—or the muscle will actually lengthen—termed eccentric activity—and power will be absorbed, and work is done on the muscle. Exercise is a potential disruption to homeostasis by these types of muscle activity which can occur exclusively or, as is more usually the case, in combination. The most important combination may be the stretch–shortening cycle, in which an eccentric action immediately precedes a concentric action. The preservation of high-force generation in the initial eccentric phase maintains the amount of elastic energy stored. During the subsequent power-generating concentric phase, the contribution of the recovered elastic energy offsets the effect of fatigue when compared to a pure concentric action.

Repeated performance of high-force eccentric actions can cause muscle damage and induces temporary muscle soreness, which is usually first felt about 6–12 h after exercise and persists for several days. The role of different fibre types in eccentric muscle activity is not well understood, although a rather small number of fibres seem to be activated to generate eccentric as compared with concentric force. There is also some evidence that Type II fibres may be selectively recruited during eccentric muscle actions. This high load on relatively few fibres may cause localized ruptures of the fibres, causing an inflammatory response with an accompanying development of swelling and pain. That muscle fibres are actually damaged is evidenced by the appearance of high levels of intramuscular enzymes in the blood in the days following the eccentric exercise bout, and histological evidence of sarcomere disruption and Z-line streaming in the affected muscles.

1.2.9 Plasticity of skeletal muscle

Skeletal muscle is a remarkably plastic tissue: it possesses a considerable capacity to adapt in response to different patterns of activity or disuse. Adaptation can take the form of alteration in muscle size, fibre composition, metabolic capacity, and capillary density. Changes in response to exercise training of an endurance and strength/power nature are dealt with in Chapter 8. Ageing has significant effects on muscle size and function (Grimby and Saltin 1983). Maximum strength of men and women is generally attained between 20 and 30 years of age. By 70 years of age, on average, the muscles are about 30% weaker. Reduced muscle mass is a primary factor in the age-associated loss of strength and may be due to a reduced muscle fibre size, particularly in the Type II fibres. There may also be an actual reduction in the total number of muscle fibres, caused by a loss of motor neurones in the elderly. Innervation of muscle fibres is required for their maintenance (possibly due to the chronic production of nerve-derived growth factors) and denervation leads to muscle fibre atrophy and eventual replacement by connective tissue. The age-associated loss of muscle mass may be caused by ageing itself, inactivity, or both. However, it is clear that muscle in the elderly still possesses the capability to adapt in response to strength training, and that significant improvements in physiological, structural, and performance characteristics can be achieved with vigorous, resistance-training programmes. As with younger adults, the frequency, intensity, and duration of exercise are crucial in determining the extent of training adaptations.

1.3 Sources of energy for muscle contraction

1.3.1 ATP

Energy is required to perform exercise and this is provided chemically in the form of ATP; in fact, energy from the hydrolysis of ATP is harnessed to provide energy for all forms of biological function. In muscle, energy from the hydrolysis of ATP by myosin ATPase activates specific sites on the force-developing elements, which allows a muscle's attempt to shorten. Active re-uptake of calcium ions by the sarcoplasmic reticulum also requires ATP. There are four mechanisms involved in the breakdown and resynthesis of ATP:

1. ATP is broken down enzymatically to adenosine diphosphate (ADP) and inorganic phosphate (P_i) to yield energy for muscle activity.
2. Phosphocreatine (PCr) is broken down enzymatically to creatine and phosphate which is transferred to ADP to re-form ATP.
3. Glucose 6-phosphate, derived from muscle glycogen or blood-borne glucose, through anaerobic glycolysis is converted to lactate and produces ATP by substrate-level phosphorylation reactions.

4. The products of carbohydrate, lipid, protein, and alcohol metabolism can enter the tricarboxylic acid (TCA or Krebs') cycle in the mitochondria and be oxidized to carbon
dioxide and water. This process is known as oxidative phosphorylation and yields
energy for the synthesis of ATP. Some of this ATP is used for the resynthesis of PCr
which becomes depleted during intense exercise.

The use of ATP as the immediate source of energy is the first of these
mechanisms, and the purpose of the other three mechanism is to regenerate ATP
at sufficient rates to prevent a significant fall in the intramuscular ATP concentration. The first three of these mechanisms, which are anaerobic (i.e. do not

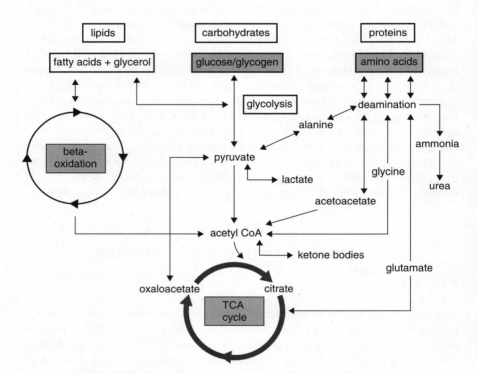

Fig. 1.7 Summary of the main pathways of energy metabolism using
carbohydrate, lipid, and protein as energy sources. Carbohydrate may participate
in both anaerobic and aerobic pathways. In glycolysis, glucose 6-phosphate
(derived from glycogen or glucose) is broken down to lactate under anaerobic
conditions and pyruvate under aerobic conditions. The pyruvate is converted to
acetyl-CoA and is completely oxidized in the TCA cycle. Lipids, in the form of
triacylglycerols, are hydrolysed to fatty acids and glycerol, the latter entering the
glycolytic pathway; fatty acids are converted via the β-oxidation pathway to
acetyl-CoA and subsequently oxidized in the TCA cycle. Protein catabolism
provides amino acids that can be converted either into TCA cycle intermediates
or into pyruvate or acetoacetate and subsequently transformed to acetyl-CoA.

use oxygen), each use only one specific substrate for energy production (i.e. ATP, PCr, and glucose 6-phosphate). Although glycerol can enter the glycolytic pathway in liver and some other tissues, it does not appear to be an energy source for skeletal muscle during exercise, probably because of the lack of the enzyme glycerol kinase in muscle.

The aerobic (oxygen using) processes in the mitochondria metabolize a variety of substrates. The sarcoplasm contains a variety of enzymes which can convert carbohydrates, lipids, and proteins into useable substrate, primarily a 2-carbon acetyl group linked to coenzyme A (acetyl-CoA) which can be completely oxidized in the mitochondria with the resultant production of ATP. A general summary of the main energy sources and pathways of energy metabolism is presented in Fig. 1.7.

1.3.2 Anaerobic metabolism

Human skeletal muscle can exert force without the use of oxygen, as a consequence of its ability to generate energy anaerobically. Two separate systems are available to the muscle to permit this, namely the phosphagen or high-energy phosphate system and the glycolytic system. Because the glycolytic system depends on the production of lactate whereas the phophagen system involves no lactate formation, these systems of anaerobic ATP regeneration are sometimes referred to as the lactate and the alactate systems, respectively. Note that the terms lactic acid and lactate are often used interchangeably, but although lactic acid is perhaps a more descriptive term, clearly indicating the acidic nature of the molecule, lactate is more accurate and will be used here. Details of these energy systems follow in Chapters 2 and 3 and only a brief overview is given here.

1.3.3 Phosphagen system

If a muscle is poisoned with cyanide and iodoacetic acid, so that it cannot derive energy from either oxidative metabolism or from the production of lactate, it can still exert force strongly for a short period of time before fatigue occurs. This tells us that the muscle has another source of energy, and also that the capacity of this energy source is limited. This source is the intramuscular store of ATP and phosphocreatine (PCr, also known as creatine phosphate)—together, ATP and PCr are referred to as the phosphagens.

The most important property of the phosphagens is that the energy store they represent is available to the muscle almost immediately. The PCr in muscle can be used to resynthesize ATP at a very high rate. This high rate of energy transfer corresponds to the ability to produce rapid forceful actions. The major disadvantage of this system is its limited capacity—the total amount of energy available is small. If no other energy source is available to the muscle, fatigue will occur rapidly. During short sprints over a distance of 30–50 m, no slowing down occurs over the last few metres—full power can be maintained all the way—and the energy requirements are met by breakdown of the phosphagen stores. Over longer distances, running speed begins to fall off as these stores become depleted and power output declines. However, the rate of recovery from a short sprint is quite rapid, and a second burst can be completed at the same speed after only 2–3 min recovery. For longer sprints (100 m or more), much longer recovery periods are needed before the ability to produce a maximum performance is restored.

1.3.4 Glycolytic system

Under normal conditions, muscle clearly does not fatigue after only a few seconds of effort, so a source of energy other than the phosphagens must be available. This is derived from glycolysis, the name given to the pathway involving the breakdown of glucose or glucose 1-phosphate, the end-product of this series of chemical reactions being pyruvate. This process does not use oxygen, but does result in energy in the form of ATP being available to the muscle from reactions involving substrate-level phosphorylation. For the reactions to proceed the pyruvate must be removed; in low-intensity exercise, when the rate at which energy is required can be met aerobically, pyruvate is converted to carbon dioxide and water by oxidative metabolism in the mitochondria. In some situations the pyruvate is removed by conversion to lactate, anaerobically, leading to the system being referred to as the lactate anaerobic system.

Activation of the glycolytic system occurs almost instantaneously at the onset of exercise, despite the number of reactions involved (for details of the glycolytic pathway see Chapter 3). The rate of lactate formation is dependent primarily on the intensity of the exercise, but depends more on the relative exercise intensity ($\%\dot{V}O_2max$) than the absolute intensity.

The total capacity of the glycolytic system for producing energy in the form of ATP is large in comparison with the phosphagen system (Table 1.2). In high-

Table 1.2   Capacity and power of anaerobic systems for the production of ATP[a]

	Capacity (mmol ATP kg dm^{-1})	Power (mmol ATP kg dm^{-1} s^{-1})
Phosphagen system	55–95	9
Glycolytic system	190–300	4.5
Combined	250–370	11

a Values are expressed per kg dry mass (dm) of muscle, and are based on estimates of ATP provision during high-intensity exercise of human vastus lateralis muscle.

intensity exercise, the muscle glycogen stores are broken down rapidly with a correspondingly high rate of lactate formation: some of the lactate diffuses out of the muscle fibres where it is produced and appears in the blood. A large part, but not all, of the muscle glycogen store can be used for anaerobic energy production during high-intensity exercise, and will supply the major part of the energy requirement for maximum-intensity efforts lasting from 20 s to 5 min. For shorter durations, the phosphagens are the major energy source, whereas oxidative metabolism becomes progressively more important as the duration (or distance) increases.

Although the total capacity of the glycolytic system is greater than that of the phosphagen system, the rate at which it can produce energy (ATP) is lower (Table 1.2). The power output that can be sustained by this system is, therefore, correspondingly lower, and it is for this reason that maximum speeds cannot be sustained for more than a few seconds—once the phosphagens are depleted, the intensity of exercise must necessarily fall.

1.3.5 Aerobic metabolism: oxidation of carbohydrate, lipid, and protein

Other pathways for regenerating ATP rely mainly on the provision of carbohydrate or lipid substrates from intramuscular stores and the circulation and their subsequent breakdown (catabolism) to yield energy to fuel substrate-level phosphorylation or the reactions of the electron transport chain and oxidative phosphorylation. To regenerate ATP from lipid (fat) catabolism, the use of oxygen is required, whereas carbohydrate catabolism can occur with or without the use of oxygen (via the glycolytic pathway described above).

The catabolism of glucose begins with anaerobic glycolysis; this yields two molecules of pyruvate (or lactate) and two molecules of ATP from each molecule of glucose that enters the glycolytic pathway (although three molecules of ATP are derived for each glucose moiety if the initial substrate is muscle glycogen). In aerobic metabolism, mostly pyruvate (rather than lactate) is formed which is converted to acetyl-CoA by the enzyme pyruvate dehydrogenase (Fig. 1.7). The catabolism of lipid in the form of fatty acids also results in the formation of acetyl-CoA (see Chapter 4 for details). Acetyl-CoA is the major fuel for the TCA cycle which occurs within the mitochondria.

In comparison to the catabolism of carbohydrate and lipid, the breakdown of protein is usually a relatively minor source of energy of exercise. In most situations, protein catabolism contributes less than 5% of the energy provision for muscle activity during physical activity. Protein catabolism can provide both ketogenic and glycogenic amino acids which may eventually be oxidized either by deamination and conversion into one of the intermediate substrates in the TCA cycle, or by conversion to pyruvic acid or acetoacetic acid and eventual transformation to acetyl-CoA (Fig. 1.7). However, during starvation and when glycogen stores become depleted, protein catabolism can become an increasingly important source of energy for exercise.

Carbohydrate, lipid, and protein catabolism will be considered in detail in subsequent chapters. However, since acetyl-CoA is a common metabolite of carbohydrate, lipid, and protein catabolism (Fig. 1.7) and the final aerobic pathways of the TCA cycle and oxidative phosphorylation are common to all three classes of fuel substrate, these important pathways of energy metabolism will be dealt with in this chapter.

1.4 Tricarboxylic acid cycle

The main function of the TCA cycle is to degrade the acetyl-CoA substrate to carbon dioxide and hydrogen atoms, and this takes place within the mitochondria (Fig. 1.8). The hydrogen atoms are then oxidized via the electron transport (respiratory) chain allowing oxidative phosphorylation with the subsequent regeneration of ATP from ADP.

As shown in Fig. 1.9, the 6-carbon tricarboxylic acid molecule citrate is formed when a 4-carbon molecule of oxaloacetate condenses with the 2-carbon acetyl group of acetyl-CoA and is subsequently hydrolysed. This reaction is catalysed by the enzyme citrate synthase. Citrate is then converted by the enzyme aconitase to its isomer isocitrate, which then undergoes oxidative decarboxylation to α-ketoglutarate. During this reaction, catalysed by isocitrate dehydrogenase, a molecule of carbon dioxide and the first of three NADH molecules produced by the TCA cycle are released while α-ketoglutarate is formed. Another molecule of carbon dioxide is released, and another NADH molecule is formed during the subsequent oxidative decarboxylation of α-ketoglutarate to form succinyl-CoA by the α-ketoglutarate dehydrogenase enzyme complex. The energy released from the breaking of the thioester (C–S) bond of succinyl-CoA is then used to phosphorylate guanosine diphosphate (GDP) thus forming guanosine triphosphate (GTP) and succinate. An enzyme called nucleotide diphosphate kinase catalyses the production of ATP by transferring the terminal phosphate group of GTP to ADP. Note that succinate is a 4-carbon compound; the original 6-carbon skeleton of the citrate molecule has undergone two decarboxylation reactions each removing a carbon atom in the form of carbon dioxide.

Succinate is subsequently oxidized to fumarate by succinate dehydrogenase and the coenzyme flavin–adenine dinucleotide (FAD), rather than NAD$^+$, is reduced to FADH$_2$. Fumarate then undergoes a hydration reaction catalysed by fumarase to form malate. The enzyme malate dehydrogenase then oxidizes the malate to form oxaloacetate with the accompanying reduction of NAD$^+$ to NADH. Note that oxaloacetate has now been re-formed and that during this one complete turn of the TCA cycle, one molecule of ATP, three molecules of

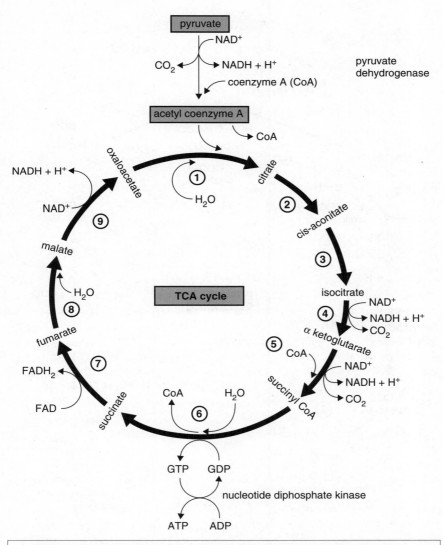

ENZYMES: **1**. Citrate synthase **2**. Aconitase **3**. Aconitase **4**. Isocitrate dehydrogenase **5**. α-Ketoglutarate dehydrogenase **6**. Succinyl CoA synthetase **7**. Succinate dehydrogenase **8**. Fumarase **9**. Malate dehydrogenase

Fig. 1.8 Summary of reactions of the tricarboxylic acid (TCA) cycle showing sites of substrate-level phosphorylation and NAD^+ and FAD reduction. α-ketoglutarate may also be referred to as 2-oxoglutarate.

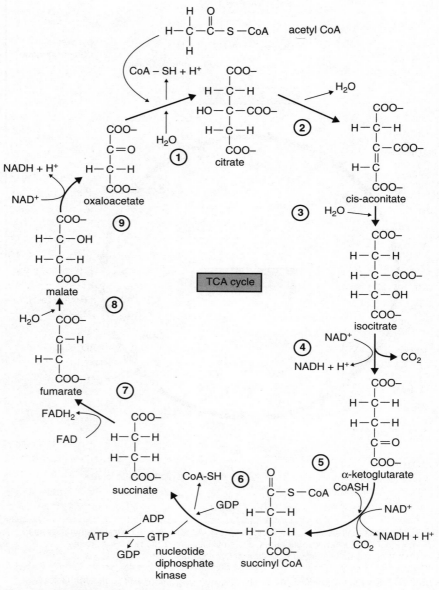

Fig. 1.9 Tricarboxylic acid (TCA) cycle.

NADH, and one of $FADH_2$ have been formed. Hence the overall reaction involving each molecule of acetyl-CoA is as follows:

$$acetyl\ CoA + ADP + 3NAD^+ + FAD \rightarrow 2CO_2 + ATP + 3NADH + 3H^+ + FADH_2CoA$$

[TCA Equation]

The 4-carbon oxaloacetate can also be formed from 3-carbon pyruvate by the enzyme pyruvate carboxylase (using the coenzyme biotin as the carrier of activated carbon dioxide) at the cost of one molecule of ATP. The activity of this enzyme is stimulated by a high concentration of acetyl-CoA, effectively signalling the need for more oxaloacetate. This reaction is important in the replenishment of TCA cycle intermediates and in the provision of substrates for gluconeogenesis, namely the formation of glucose from non-carbohydrate precursors.

A key regulatory point in the TCA cycle is the reaction catalysed by citrate synthase. The activity of this enzyme is inhibited by ATP, NADH, succinyl-CoA, and acyl-CoA derivatives of fatty acids; the activity of the enzyme is also affected by citrate availability. Hence, when cellular energy levels are high, flux through the TCA cycle is relatively low, but this can be greatly increased when ATP and NADH utilization is increased, as during exercise.

Note that molecular oxygen does not participate directly in the reactions of the TCA cycle. In essence, the most important function of the TCA cycle is to generate hydrogen atoms for their subsequent passage to the electron transport chain by means of NAD^+ and FAD (Fig. 1.10). The aerobic process of electron transport–oxidative phosphorylation regenerates ATP from ADP, thus conserving some of the chemical energy contained within the original substrates in the form of high-energy phosphates. As long as there is an adequate supply of O_2 and substrate is available, NAD^+ and FAD are continuously regenerated and TCA metabolism proceeds.

1.5 Electron transport chain

The electron transport chain (Fig. 1.11) represents a series of linked carrier molecules which remove electrons from hydrogen and eventually pass them to molecular oxygen; oxygen also accepts hydrogen to form water. Much of the energy generated in the transfer of electrons from hydrogen to oxygen is trapped or conserved as chemical potential energy in the form of high-energy phosphates; the remainder is lost as heat. During the previously mentioned dehydrogenase reactions of the TCA cycle (and glycolysis), NAD^+ is reduced and gains a hydrogen and two electrons; the other hydrogen appears in the intracellular fluid as H^+. FAD is the other coenzyme that is reduced in dehydrogenation reactions and this also accepts pairs of electrons; FAD also accepts both hydrogen atoms to become $FADH_2$. NADH and $FADH_2$ are energy-rich molecules

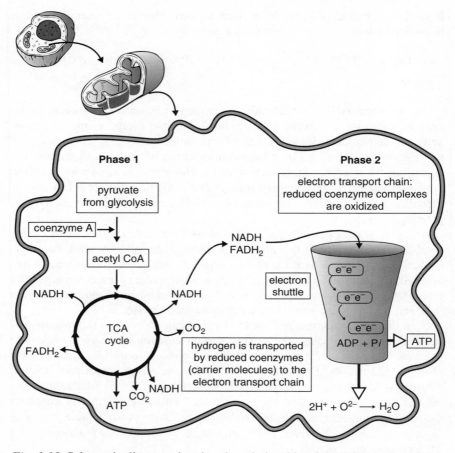

Fig. 1.10 Schematic diagram showing the relationship of the TCA cycle to the electron transport chain.

because they each contain a pair of electrons that have a high energy-transfer potential. During the process of transferring these electrons to oxygen, a large amount of energy is liberated which can be used to phosphorylate ADP, thus regenerating ATP. The transport of electrons from NADH and $FADH_2$ to molecular oxygen is accomplished by a series of specific carriers located on the inner membrane of mitochondria; these carriers constitute the electron transport or respiratory chain.

In the first step of the electron transport chain, catalysed by an NADH dehydrogenase enzyme complex, two electrons are transferred from NADH to flavin mononucleotide (FMN) to form $FMNH_2$, and energy released during this transfer of electrons is used to phosphorylate ADP (ATP synthesis site #1 in Fig. 1.11). The electrons are then transferred to coenzyme Q (CoQ) which is

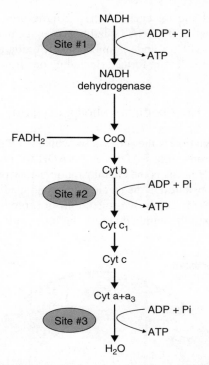

Fig. 1.11 Electron transport chain showing the sites of ATP synthesis.

also capable of accepting electrons from $FADH_2$; thus, $FADH_2$ enters the electron transport chain beyond the first site of ATP synthesis. Note the reason for this is that the $FADH_2$ exists at a lower energy state than NADH and $FMNH_2$, so that FMN cannot accept electrons from $FADH_2$. Following CoQ, the remaining electron carriers in the respiratory chain are haem (iron) - containing proteins called cytochromes. Each cytochrome can carry only one electron (rather than two as with NADH, $FMNH_2$, and $CoQH_2$). The iron moiety of each cytochrome can exist in either its oxidized ferric (Fe^{3+}) form or reduced ferrous (Fe^{2+}) form. By accepting an electron, the ferric iron of a specific cytochrome becomes reduced to its ferrous form. In turn, this donates its electron to the next cytochrome down the line, and the last one, cytochrome a_3, discharges its electron directly to molecular oxygen.

Electrons are passed from CoQ to cytochrome b and then to cytochrome c_1, at which point another ATP molecule is synthesized (site #2 in Fig. 1.11). Electrons are transferred from cytochrome c_1 to cytochrome c, and then on to cytochromes a and a_3 which exist as a complex called cytochrome oxidase. Cytochrome a_3 finally transfers the electrons to molecular oxygen and a third ATP molecule is synthesized at this point (site #3 in Fig. 1.11). Hence, for each molecule of NADH that enters the electron transport chain, three molecules of

ATP are regenerated and for each $FADH_2$, 2 molecules of ATP are formed. Thus, by referring back to the TCA Equation above, it can be calculated that for each molecule of acetyl-CoA undergoing complete oxidation in the TCA cycle, a total of 12 ATP molecules are formed (including one from GTP).

1.6 Oxidative phosphorylation

Oxidative phosphorylation is the process by which ATP is synthesized during the transfer of electrons from $FADH_2$ and NADH to molecular oxygen. The accepted mechanism for this is the chemiosmotic theory proposed by Mitchell: the transfer of electrons through the electron transport chain located on the inner mitochondrial membrane causes hydrogen ions or protons (H^+) from the inner mitochondrial matrix to be pumped across the inner mitochondrial membrane

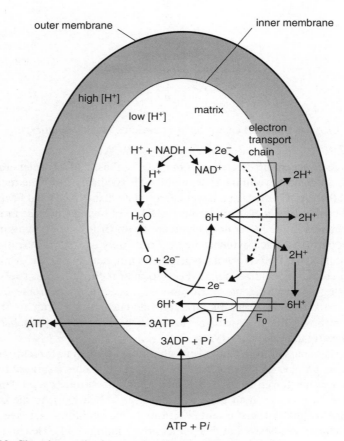

Fig. 1.12 Chemiosmotic theory of oxidative phosphorylation.

into the space between the inner and outer mitochondrial membranes, Fig. 1.12). The high concentration of positively charged hydrogen ions in this outer chamber causes the H^+ ions to flow back into the mitochondrial matrix through the F_0–F_1 protein complex embedded in the inner mitochondrial membrane. The flow of H^+ ions (protons) through this complex constitutes a proton-motive force that is used to drive ATP synthesis. The F_0 subunit of the complex is the proton channel and the F_1 subunit is the coupling unit that contains ATP synthase activity.

1.7 Carbohydrate and lipid stores

Carbohydrates are stored in the body as a glucose polymer called glycogen. Skeletal muscle contains a significant store of glycogen in the sarcoplasm. The glycogen content of skeletal muscle at rest is approximately 14–18 g per kg wet mass (80–100 mmol glucosyl units kg^{-1}). The liver also contains glycogen; about 80–110 g are stored in the liver of an adult human in the post-absorptive state, which can be released into the circulation in order to maintain the blood glucose concentration at about 5 $mmol^{-2}$ (0.9 g per litre). Lipids are stored as triglyceride (triacylglycerol), mainly in white adipose tissue. This must first be broken down by a lipase (fat-splitting) enzyme to release free fatty acids (FFA) into the circulation for uptake by working muscle. Skeletal muscle also contains some triacylglycerol which can be used as an energy source during exercise following lipolysis, and this source of fuel may become relatively more important after exercise training. Lipid stores in the body are far larger than those of carbohydrate and lipid is a more efficient storage form of energy, releasing 37 kJ g^{-1} compared with 16 kJ g^{-1} of carbohydrate. Each gram of carbohydrate stored also retains about 3 g of water, thus further decreasing the efficiency of carbohydrate as an energy source. The energy cost of running a marathon is about 12 000 kJ; if this could be achieved by the oxidation of fat alone, the total amount of lipid required would be about 320 g, whereas 750 g of carbohydrate and an additional 2.3 kg of associated water would be required if carbohydrate oxidation were the sole source of energy. Apart from considerations of the weight to be carried, this amount of carbohydrate exceeds the total amount normally stored in the liver, muscles and blood combined. The total storage capacity for lipid is extremely large, and for most practical purposes the amount of energy stored in the form of fat is far in excess of that required for any exercise task (Table 1.3).

Protein is not stored, other than as functionally important molecules (e.g. structural proteins, enzymes, ion channels, receptors, contractile proteins, etc.), and the concentration of most free amino acids in intracellular and extracellular body fluids is quite low. It is not surprising then that, in most situations, carbohydrate and lipids supply most of the energy required to regenerate ATP to fuel exercise.

Table 1.3   Energy stores in the average man[a]

	Weight (g)	Energy (kJ)
Liver glycogen	80	1280
Muscle glycogen	350	5600
Blood glucose	10	160
Lipid	10 500	388 500
Protein	12 000	204 000

a This assumes a body weight of 70 kg and a fat content of 15% of body weight. The value for blood glucose includes the glucose content of extracellular fluid. Not all of this, and not more than a very small part of the total protein, is available for use during exercise.

1.8 Methods of estimating substrate use

A number of different methods have been used to study energy metabolism in both animals and humans. The respiratory exchange ratio (RER) during steady-state conditions can give a reasonable estimate of the proportions of carbohydrate and lipid being oxidized: an RER of 1.0 indicates that only carbohydrate is being oxidized, whereas an RER of 0.7 indicates that fat is the sole substrate being oxidized. The RER in the post-absorptive state at rest is usually about 0.8. However, the RER, which is measured at the mouth, is only an indirect measure of the respiratory quotient (RQ) which is the actual ratio of the production of carbon dioxide and utilization of oxygen at the cellular level (and, therefore, the most accurate reflection of the substrate mixture being used). Even so, several studies have been able to confirm that the RER is reasonably representative of the RQ, provided that a steady state exists in the ventilation and acid–base balance. Hyperventilation during exercise may blow off additional carbon dioxide and increase the RER. Lactic acid accumulation in the blood will form additional carbon dioxide from bicarbonate and further stimulate ventilation, producing an RER greater than 1.0. In this case, it is common to assume that the RER is 1.0 and that carbohydrate is the main fuel; this assumption is reasonable given that lactate accumulation and hyperventilation will only normally occur at fairly high intensities of dynamic exercise (i.e. > 80% $\dot{V}O_2$max) when individuals may also never reach a steady state.

Other methods rely on the sampling of tissue and blood, before, during, and after exercise. Blood samples can be used to determine the circulating concentrations of fuel substrates such as glucose, triacylglycerol, free fatty acids, glycerol, ketone bodies, and amino acids. However, concentration measurements in blood do not necessarily reveal all about the turnover rate: for example, a glucose molecule in the blood has a half-life of only a few minutes. However, the measurement of blood flow rate and simultaneous sampling of arterial and venous blood can give a measure of tissue uptake or release of a particular substrate. Radioactive or naturally labelled isotopes of ingested or injected substances such as glucose, fatty acids, or amino acids will reveal their rates of uptake, oxidation, or clearance when expired gases, blood, or urine are analysed.

Biopsy samples of muscle can be used to determine intramuscular concentrations of energy reserves (e.g. glycogen, triacylglycerols) and metabolic intermediates, and can also be used to provide information on fibre type composition, capillary and mitochondrial densities, and the activities of various enzymes. *In vitro* studies of muscle samples also allow the estimation of maximum metabolic capacities for the oxidation of various substrates.

Recently developed microdialysis techniques applied to muscle and adipose tissue allow the estimation of substrate and metabolite exchange between the interstitial fluid and the surrounding tissue. For example, the release of glycerol into the interstitial fluid in adipose tissue is thought to provide a good indication of the rate of lipolysis. The main limitation to this particular technique is the time required (at least several minutes) for the collection of a sufficient volume of dialysis fluid for metabolite analysis.

Other techniques can study substrate use directly in the body. For example, the magnetic resonance spectroscopy (MRS) technique can be used to estimate changes in the concentrations of high-energy phosphates and glycogen (and pH) in muscle and positron emission tomography (PET) can be used to reveal glucose metabolism in the brain.

1.9 Factors influencing the utilization of fuel sources during exercise

A number of factors are known to influence the selection of fuel for exercise, and there can be significant interactions between several of them. These factors include: substrate availability; nutritional status; diet; mode, intensity, and duration of exercise; muscle fibre type composition; physical fitness; or the effect of: training; drugs; hormones; prior exercise; and environmental factors such as temperature and altitude. The main factors influencing substrate use during exercise are summarized in Table 1.4. These are mostly dealt with in some detail in following chapters.

1.9.1 Intensity and duration of exercise

The most important factor influencing the selection of fuel for muscular work is the intensity of exercise. Table 1.5 represents the proportions of the energy demand for a given level of fatiguing exercise over different exercise durations that are derived from anaerobic or aerobic sources. For example, in a 100 m sprint, run in about 10 s, about 90% of the energy is derived from anaerobic

Table 1.4 Factors influencing substrate utilization during exercise

1. *Substrate availability*
   Glycogen and lipid stores in muscle
   Glucose release from liver into blood
   Lipolysis in adipose tissue, releasing free fatty acids into blood
   Blood flow rate in muscle
   Amino acids in muscle
2. *Oxygen availability*
   For electron transport and oxidative phosphorylation
3. *Activity of rate-limiting enzymes*
   Concentration
   Balance between inhibitors and activators
   Feedback control
   Effects of changes in muscle pH
4. *Levels of plasma hormones*

NB: These in turn are affected by a number of important influences including:
1. Previous exercise and diet
2. Muscle fibre composition
3. Type, intensity, and duration of exercise
4. Exercise training
5. Environment (temperature, humidity, altitude)
6. Drugs (e.g. caffeine)

Table 1.5 Approximate contribution of aerobic and anaerobic energy sources to total energy production in events of different durations involving maximal work

Distance	Duration[a] (min: s)	% Aerobic	% Anaerobic
100 m	9.84	10	90
400 m	43.29	30	70
800 m	1 : 41.73	60	40
1500 m	3 : 27.37	80	20
5000 m	12 : 44.39	95	5
10 000 m	26 : 38.08	97	3
42.2 km	126 : 50	99	1

a Durations given are the current men's outdoor world records at 1 April 1997.

sources. For the marathon, run over a distance of 42.2 km in just under 127 min (current world record), 99% of the energy expended is derived from aerobic sources. Thus, the oxygen supply to the muscles, which is dependent on the exercise intensity and the duration following exercise onset, is a major determining factor of substrate use.

1.9.2 Muscle fibre type composition

A number of cross-sectional studies have shown that élite endurance athletes possess a greater percentage of slow-twitch Type I fibres than do sprinters, who possess a greater percentage of Type II fibres. As mentioned earlier, the fibre-type metabolic characteristics have a major influence on the ability of an individual to develop a high-power output or sustain exercise for a prolonged period of time. Thus, the fibre-type composition is a determinant of the absolute intensity and duration of exercise that can be performed by an individual, which, in turn, are two of the primary factors determining substrate use.

1.9.3 Diet and feeding during exercise

The proportions of fat and carbohydrate in the diet and the intake of carbohydrate during exercise can significantly influence substrate availability and utilization. Substrate availability is a major factor in influencing the selection of fuel for exercise. High-carbohydrate diets will maintain or raise the muscle and liver glycogen content and also increase the proportion of energy derived from carbohydrate during exercise. Starvation and high-fat (low-carbohydrate) diets elevate the plasma FFA concentration, which is a determining factor in their rate of utilization and will increase the relative contribution of lipid to oxidative metabolism.

Many of the coenzymes in the energy metabolic pathways are derivatives of vitamins which cannot be synthesized in the body. Deficiencies of such vitamins impair exercise performance and influence substrate utilization. Vitamin B_{12} and folic acid are required for the normal production of red blood cells (erythrocytes) in the bone marrow; deficiencies of these can impair the oxygen-carrying capacity of the blood, necessitating an increased reliance on anaerobic fuel sources during exercise. Minerals are also important. For example, iron is an essential component of haemoglobin, the oxygen-carrying pigment of the red blood cells, so an iron deficiency can impair the ability of the blood to transport oxygen.

1.9.4 Exercise training

Training adaptations in muscle also affect substrate utilization. Endurance training increases the mitochondrial density of muscle (an effect that is specific to the muscles used in the training activity), increases capillary density, increases the relative cross-sectional area of Type I fibres, increases intramuscular content of triacylglycerol, and increases the capacity to use lipid as an energy source during submaximal intensities of exercise. Trained subjects also demonstrate an increased reliance on intramuscular lipid as an energy source during exercise.

These effects, and other physiological effects of training (improved oxygen delivery to working muscle and altered hormonal responses to exercise), decrease the rate of utilization of muscle glycogen and blood glucose and decrease the rate of accumulation of lactate during submaximal exercise. These adaptations contribute to the marked improvement in endurance capacity following training.

1.9.5 Prior exercise

Prior exercise of sufficient intensity and duration to deplete glycogen stores, coupled with insufficient recovery time (say less than 24 h) to restore the glycogen concentration to pre-exercise levels can decrease carbohydrate utilization, with an increase in lipid utilization, during exercise performed on subsequent days.

1.9.6 Drugs

Some drugs have marked effects on substrate availability and utilization during exercise. A classic example is caffeine, which increases the mobilization of FFA from adipose tissue and hence elevates the plasma FFA concentration. Since during the first 30 min or so of exercise at about 70% $\dot{V}O_2$max, plasma FFA concentration is slow to increase (or may initially decrease), the ingestion of caffeine in sufficient dosage to markedly elevate lipolysis and raise the plasma FFA availability in the early stages of exercise can spare the utilization of the limited stores of muscle glycogen, allowing exercise to be sustained for longer. Caffeine is also known to have neurological effects, which may be more important for its ergogenic effect. Other procedures which raise the plasma FFA concentration (e.g. intravenous injection of heparin) also increase the contribution of fat oxidation to energy provision and result in glycogen sparing. Administration of nicotinic acid, which inhibits lipolysis, has the opposite effect. Other drugs influence substrate utilization by altering hormonal responses to exercise or by acting as agonists or antagonists to hormone actions.

1.9.7 Hormones

Many hormones influence energy metabolism in the body (for a detailed review see Galbo 1983). During exercise, interactions between insulin, glucagon, and the catecholamines (adrenaline and noradrenaline) are mostly responsible for fuel substrate availability and utilization; cortisol and growth hormone also have some significant effects. A summary of the hormone and metabolite regulation of ATP replenishment via anaerobic and aerobic pathways during exercise is

Table 1.6a   Summary of the regulation of anaerobic ATP replenishment pathways by hormones and metabolites during exercise

---

Activation of PCr breakdown
1. Decreased ratio of ATP:ADP because of ATP breakdown during muscle contraction

Inhibition of PCr breakdown
1. Increased ratio of ATP:ADP due to increased aerobic production of ATP or decreased rate of ATP utilization because of fall in power output

Activation of glycolysis
1. Decreased ratio of ATP:(ADP + AMP) because of ATP breakdown during muscle contraction
2. Decreased concentration of PCr because it is used to buffer ATP stores during contraction
3. Increased calcium ion concentration because it is released from the sarcoplasmic reticulum during contraction
4. Increased circulating levels of adrenaline (from adrenal glands) and noradrenaline (mainly from sympathetic nerve endings) activating phosphorylase
5. Increased fructose 6-phosphate concentration

Inhibition of glycolysis
1. Increased ratio of ATP:(ADP + AMP) because of increased aerobic production of ATP or decreased rate of ATP utilization due to a fall in power output
2. Increased citrate concentration mainly resulting from increased FFA and acetyl CoA catabolism via the TCA cycle
3. Increased concentration of PCr because it is replenished by aerobic ATP production or if the power output falls
4. Decreased calcium ion concentration in sarcoplasm during relaxation
5. Reduced pH resulting from lactic acid accumulation
6. Increased FFA concentration, which inhibits glucose entry into muscle

---

presented in Tables 1.6*a* and *b*. Further details are provided in subsequent chapters.

1.9.8 Environmental factors

High environmental temperatures and dehydration are detrimental to exercise performance and influence substrate utilization during exercise. An elevated rate of utilization of muscle glycogen has been reported during exercise at 70–85% $\dot{V}O_2$max in the heat (41 °C), together with a higher blood lactate concentration. These effects could be due to a shift of blood flow to the skin and a reduced blood volume contributing to a reduced perfusion of exercising muscle. The decreased oxygen (and substrate) delivery to muscle leads to a greater reliance on carbohydrate to sustain the required exercise intensity, both aerobically and

Table 1.6b   Summary of the regulation of aerobic ATP replenishment pathways by hormones and metabolites during exercise

---

Activation of FFA oxidation
1.   Increased plasma FFA concentration because of greater mobilization of FFA from adipose tissue due to: (a) elevated circulating levels of adrenaline, noradrenaline, glucagon, growth hormone, and cortisol; and (b) decreased circulating level of insulin

Inhibition of FFA oxidation
1.   Increased blood lactate accumulation during heavy exercise inhibiting lipolysis
2.   Increased insulin concentration after carbohydrate consumption

Activation of oxidative phosphorylation
1.   Increased mitochondrial ADP concentration due to ATP breakdown during muscle contraction
2.   Increased delivery of oxygen to the mitochondria

Inhibition of oxidative phosphorylation
1.   Decreased mitochondrial ADP concentration as ATP is regenerated via the electron transport chain or if power output falls
2.   Decreased oxygen availability to the mitochondria
3.   Decreased availability of NADH and $FADH_2$ as TCA cycle activity declines

---

anaerobically. Exercise at altitude, where the ambient partial pressure of oxygen is lower than at sea level, will also reduce oxygen delivery to working muscle and result in an increased contribution from carbohydrate and anaerobic energy sources during intense exercise.

1.10   Delivery of blood-borne fuel and oxygen to muscle during exercise

The availability of extramuscular fuel and of oxygen influence metabolic responses to exercise. Cardiovascular and pulmonary physiology is therefore highly relevant to any consideration of muscle metabolism during different intensities and durations of exercise performed under varying environmental conditions. The following discussion aims to give a brief overview of cardiovascular and pulmonary responses to exercise and the factors that influence muscle blood flow and oxygen uptake.

1.10.1 Blood flow distribution

At rest, the rate of blood flow to human skeletal muscle is about 20–30 ml min^{-1} kg muscle^{-1} and the effective (open) capillary density is about 100 per mm^2.

Tonic sympathetic tone maintains constriction of many arterioles and the majority of the capillaries are not perfused.

During exercise, despite an increase in sympathetic nervous activity, the blood vessels in active muscle dilate and the effective capillary density is increased up to five-fold compared with rest. The exercise-induced vasodilation of the active muscular vasculature is brought about by local factors arising from the increased metabolism in the contracting muscles. These local factors include a fall in pO_2, a rise in pCO_2, decreased pH, elevated temperature, and increases in the concentrations of adenosine, nitric oxide, P_i, and potassium in the extra-cellular fluid. This localized vasodilation to exercising muscle (inactive muscles undergo vasoconstriction) during exercise, together with an increased cardiac output, allow an increased rate of blood flow to the active muscles which can be up to 100-fold greater than at rest. Not only does the active musculature receive a greater blood flow during exercise, it also receives a greater proportion of the (increased) cardiac output compared with rest (Fig. 1.13). Recent work has shown that the increase in muscle blood flow during exercise is almost instant-aneous and that it plateaus very quickly. This implies that the limit to the oxygen consumption in the early stages of exercise (i.e. during the non-steady-state period) is not oxygen delivery to the working muscle.

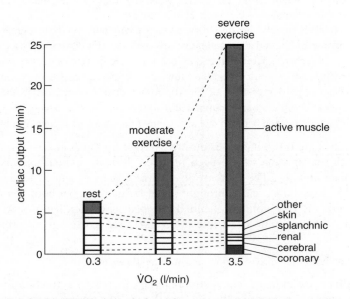

Fig. 1.13 Regional distribution of blood flow at rest and during two intensities of exercise.

1.10.2 Cardiac output and venous return

[handwritten margin notes: Homeostasis / why is a lise / a lise]

The cardiac output at rest is about 5–6 litres min^{-1} in an adult human. The cardiac output must increase during exercise to supply the increased demand for blood flow by the working muscles. However, an increased output of blood pumped from the heart can only be achieved if the venous return of blood from the tissues to the right side of the heart is increased. Furthermore, arterial blood pressure (BP) must also be maintained: a substantial vasodilation of the active muscle vasculature would decrease peripheral resistance and cause a drastic fall in arterial BP if not compensated for by other effects. Peripheral resistance is maintained and venous return increased during exercise due to a number of effects:

1. A generalized vasoconstriction resulting from increased sympathetic nervous activity (sympathetic nerves innervate arterioles and cause contraction of the smooth muscle in their walls, hence constricting their diameter when sympathetic activity is increased).
2. A generalized constriction of the veins. These are the capacitance vessels of the circulation. At rest about 65% of the total blood volume is present in the veins. Some of this volume can be shunted to the arterial side of the circulation by constriction (reduction in diameter and stiffening) of the walls of the major veins.
3. The contraction of the muscles of the limbs (particularly the legs) compresses the veins that run in parallel through the muscle tissue. This causes a pumping action which speeds the return of blood to the thorax. Valves in the veins prevent any backflow of blood during the phases when the limb muscles relax. This effect is sometimes referred to as the 'skeletal muscle pump'.
4. During inspiration the pressure in the thoracic cavity falls. As the diaphragm contracts during inspiration, it flattens and moves downwards. This causes a slight compression of the abdomen, increasing abdominal pressure, compressing the veins in the abdomen, and hence driving blood towards the thorax (again, valves in the veins prevent the retrograde flow of blood). Although this effect, called the 'thoraco-abdominal pump', is fairly minimal at rest, it becomes of considerable significance during exercise when both the rate and depth of breathing are increased substantially.

[handwritten margin note: What lise]

Cardiac output ($\dot{Q}$) increases during exercise up to about 25–30 litres min^{-1}, although higher values have been reported during maximal exercise in élite endurance athletes. The increase in cardiac output is related to the exercise intensity (Fig. 1.14), and is brought about by increases in both heart rate and stroke volume (the volume of blood pumped with each heart beat). In adult humans, the maximum heart rate is inversely related to age according to the relationship:

Maximum heart rate = 210 − (0.65 × age in years) (beats min^{-1}).

[handwritten margin note: cause of lise]

The increase in heart rate is stimulated by increased activation of the sympathetic nerves innervating the sino-atrial node (the intrinsic pacemaker) of the heart and withdrawal of the inhibitory parasympathetic nervous activity con-

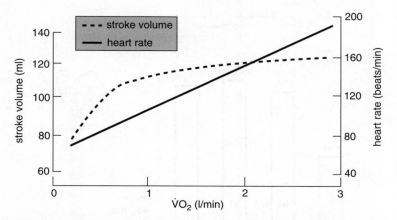

Fig. 1.14 Changes in heart rate, and stroke volume with increasing exercise intensity.

veyed via the vagus nerves. Circulating catecholamines also stimulate the heart rate. Stroke volume is increased from about 70 ml at rest to about 120 ml during exercise at 50% $\dot{V}O_2$max, with no further increase in stroke volume at higher exercise intensities. The increased stroke volume is achieved by greater filling (higher end-diastolic volume) during the relaxation phase of the cardiac cycle (diastole) and stronger contraction of the myocardium, and hence greater empty-ing of the ventricles during the contraction phase (systole) compared with rest (Fig. 1.15).

During prolonged exercise, particularly in a hot environment, there tends to be an upward drift in heart rate and a decline in stroke volume as exercise pro-gresses. This is probably caused by a reduction in the central blood volume and venous pressure as more blood gets diverted to the skin blood vessels in order to increase heat loss. Sweat losses and a fall in plasma volume also contribute to this effect.

Temp steady State.

1.10.3 Blood volume

Blood volume tends to fall slightly during exercise due mainly to a loss of plasma volume, which can be up to about 20% during very intense exercise. This loss of plasma volume results from an osmotic movement of water into active muscle. The osmolarity of the muscle sarcoplasm and interstitial fluid increases because of the breakdown and metabolism of large molecules of glycogen into many smaller molecules (e.g. pyruvate and lactate). Also the increased perfusion of capillary beds in active muscle increases the capillary hydrostatic pressure which increases the formation of interstitial fluid from plasma. To some extent, this effect is offset by a movement of fluid into the

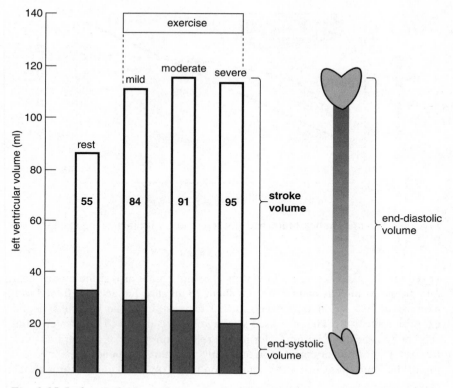

Fig. 1.15 Left ventricular volume at rest and during different intensities of exercise measured by radionuclide scintigraphy (data from Poliner *et al.* 1980).

circulation from tissues that undergo vasoconstriction (e.g. gut, liver, and kidneys) during exercise. The extent of reduction in plasma volume is directly related to the relative exercise intensity ($\dot{V}O_2$max). At an exercise intensity of 70% $\dot{V}O_2$max, plasma volume falls by about 10–15% within the first few minutes of exercise, and may be partially restored as exercise duration progresses, although this will depend on the rate of oral consumption of fluid (if any) during exercise and sweat loss influenced by the ambient temperature and humidity. The overall effect of a net loss of plasma volume is an increase in the red blood cell count and haemoglobin concentration, increasing the oxygen-carrying capacity per litre of blood, but at the expense of a reduction in total blood volume and an increase in blood viscosity.

1.10.4 Blood pressure

Mean arterial blood pressure tends to remain about the same, or slightly increases, during most forms of exercise. Substantial increases in systolic BP occur (from about 120 mmHg at rest to about 180 mmHg) during dynamic exercise because of the ejection of a larger volume of blood from the heart in a shorter time into the aorta. However, diastolic BP tends to fall slightly during exercise. Diastolic BP reflects the balance between the increased cardiac output and decreased peripheral resistance caused by the marked vasodilation of the active skeletal muscle vasculature. Typically, diastolic BP is about 80 mmHg at rest and is 60–80 mmHg during dynamic exercise. In static (isometric) efforts, both the systolic and diastolic BP rise substantially, despite only relatively small increases in cardiac output. This is because the intramuscular pressure in the active muscle during a sustained strong isometric contraction actually exceeds the systolic BP. Thus, there is little or no blood flow into the active muscle, but a marked sympathetically mediated vasoconstriction occurs in other vascular beds (except the heart and brain) which results in elevated peripheral resistance and hence a rise in both systolic and diastolic BP. It follows that the energy to fuel sustained isometric contractions is largely derived from anaerobic sources.

1.10.5 Pulmonary ventilation

Exercise markedly increases the oxygen consumption and carbon dioxide production by muscle. Hence, the pO_2 of venous blood draining active muscle is lower than at rest, and the pCO_2 is higher. The mixed venous blood pumped to the lungs from the right ventricle of the heart will also reflect this alteration in venous blood gas composition. Together with an increase in cardiac output during exercise, this causes a greater uptake of oxygen across the alveolar respiratory membrane and a greater excretion of carbon dioxide across the same. Ventilation of the lungs increases during exercise and is closely coupled to the metabolic rate that is proportional to the rate of carbon dioxide production. Thus, during light and moderate exercise (up to about 55% $\dot{V}O_2max$), ventilation increases linearly with oxygen consumption (Fig. 1.16) and carbon dioxide production, and averages 20–25 litres of air for each litre of oxygen consumed. Under these conditions, increases in ventilation are mainly achieved by increasing the tidal volume (depth of breathing), whereas at higher exercise intensities, increases in breathing frequency become relatively more important (Fig. 1.17). With this adjustment in ventilation, there is complete oxygenation of the blood because the alveolar (and arterial) pO_2 and pCO_2 remain close to resting values. In more strenuous exercise, hydrogen ions released from active muscle are first buffered by the bicarbonate (or hydrogen carbonate, HCO_3^-) present in plasma, thus releasing more CO_2, and as more hydrogen (and lactate) ions accumulate the blood pH falls. These effects provide an additional stimulus to ventilation, so that minute ventilation increases disproportionately with increases in oxygen consumption (Fig. 1.15). At work-rates close to $\dot{V}O_2max$, up to 40 litres of air may be ventilated for each litre of oxygen consumed. As a result, more CO_2 is excreted and the RER will rise above 1.0.

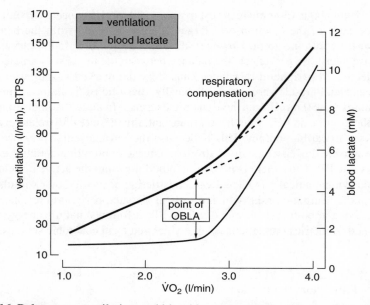

Fig. 1.16 Pulmonary ventilation and blood lactate concentration in relation to oxygen consumption during incremental exercise to the maximal oxygen uptake. The dashed line represents the extrapolation of the linear relationship between ventilation and oxygen consumption observed during low–moderate submaximal exercise intensities.

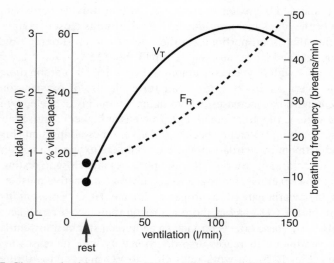

Fig. 1.17 Changes in tidal volume (V_T) and breathing frequency (F_R) with increasing intensities of exercise.

1.10.6 Blood oxygen-carrying capacity

The capacity of blood to carry oxygen is primarily determined by its haemo-globin concentration and the pO_2. When fully saturated with oxygen (which occurs at a pO_2 of about 90 mmHg or higher), each gram of haemoglobin (exclusively located in the red blood cells) can transport 1.34 ml of oxygen. Thus, for a typical man with a blood haemoglobin concentration of 150 g l^{-1}, the oxygen-carrying capacity of arterial blood is about 200 ml O_2, per litre of blood. Note that the haemoglobin concentration of the blood of females is about 10% less, and consequently so is their oxygen-carrying capacity. Oxygen is released from haemoglobin as the blood passes through the capillary beds of the tissues. The affinity of haemoglobin for oxygen is related to the pO_2, and in the capillar-ies where the pO_2 is lower (typically about 40 mmHg) than in arterial blood because of oxygen uptake by the tissues, some (about 25%) of the oxygen disso-ciates from haemoglobin and is, therefore, made available for tissue uptake (Fig. 1.18). Other factors also influence the affinity of haemoglobin for oxygen.

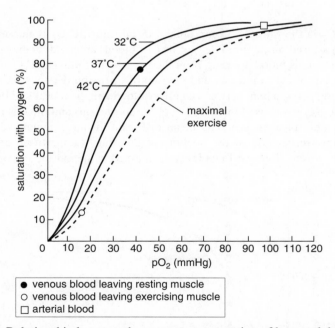

Fig. 1.18 Relationship between the percentage saturation of haemoglobin with oxygen and the partial pressure of oxygen. Note that the pO_2 in the tissue capillaries is about 40 mmHg, whereas in the pulmonary capillaries it is close to 100 mmHg. Increased temperature, pCO_2 and hydrogen ion concentration decrease the affinity of haemoglobin for oxygen at any given pO_2, effectively shifting the dissociation curve to the right. This allows greater unloading of oxygen from haemoglobin at the pO_2 in the tissue capillary beds.

Increases in pCO_2, temperature, and hydrogen ion concentration all reduce the affinity of haemoglobin for oxygen, so that at any given pO_2 more oxygen is given up to the tissues (Fig. 1.18). Such changes, of course, occur in metabolically active muscle during exercise. This effectively means that the increased oxygen demand of contracting muscle is automatically met by increased unloading of oxygen from the blood, while still largely maintaining a high pO_2 gradient from blood to the muscle mitochondria (where the pO_2 is very low, possibly as low as 1 mmHg). Maintenance of a large pO_2 gradient allows rapid diffusion to take place.

1.11 Oxygen uptake by muscle during exercise

The oxygen consumption of muscle during rest or exercise depends on the blood flow rate and the amount of oxygen that can be extracted by the tissue per litre of blood. This can be expressed as the Fick equation:

$$\dot{V}O_2 = \dot{Q} \times (C_aO_2 - C_vO_2).$$

Where $\dot{V}O_2$ is the rate of oxygen uptake in ml min^{-1}, C_aO_2 is the content of oxygen in arterial blood (in ml O_2 per litre of blood) and C_vO_2 is the content of oxygen in venous blood draining from the tissue (same units as C_aO_2). Oxygen diffuses from blood to muscle, and the rate of diffusion depends on the magnitude of the pO_2 gradient between capillary blood and the muscle mitochondria (where the oxygen is used in oxidative phosphorylation) and the distance over which oxygen must diffuse. The mean diffusion distance actually decreases during exercise because of the opening of previously unperfused capillaries around the muscle fibres. A low pO_2 is maintained in the muscle sarcoplasm by

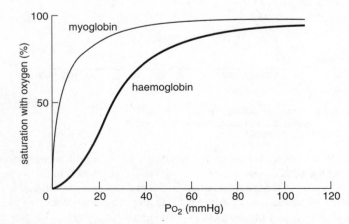

Fig. 1.19 Comparison of the oxygen dissociation curves of myoglobin and haemoglobin.

another oxygen-binding pigment called myoglobin. This pigment has a much greater affinity for oxygen than haemoglobin, and only releases oxygen at very low pO_2 (Fig. 1.19), a little above that found close to the metabolically active mitochondria. The mitochondria are not uniformly distributed within the muscle fibre, but are concentrated near to the periphery, closest to the capillaries.

During maximal exercise, muscle does not appear to be capable of extracting all the oxygen that is delivered to it by the arterial circulation; that is to say, the venous blood draining maximally active muscle is not completely desaturated of its oxygen. The percentage saturation of haemoglobin with oxygen in venous blood leaving muscle falls from about 50–60% at rest to as low as 10% during intense exercise (Fig. 1.20). The corresponding venous pO_2 is about 25–40 mmHg and 10–15 mmHg, respectively, so at high oxygen uptakes the muscles do extract most (but not all) of the oxygen delivered to them.

1.11.1 Limitations to oxygen uptake during exercise

Many factors, both physiological and pathological, can potentially limit the maximal oxygen uptake that can be attained during exercise. These are listed in Table 1.7, and can be grouped into central (pulmonary and central cardio-vascular) and peripheral (local circulatory and muscular) mechanisms.

Endurance athletes are known to have a high $\dot{V}O_2$max, and attributes which contribute to this capability have been extensively studied. To achieve a high oxygen consumption, an effective system for the transfer of oxygen from the

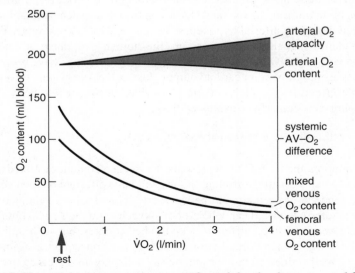

Fig. 1.20 Changes in the oxygen content of arterial, mixed venous, and femoral venous blood during increasing intensities of leg exercise.

Table 1.7   Possible limitations to maximal oxygen consumption during exercise

Central limitations

1. *Respiratory*
   (a) Ventilation
   (b) Alveolar ventilation
   (c) Oxygen diffusion

   (d) Affinity of haemoglobin for oxygen

2. *Central circulation*
   (a) Cardiac output
   (b) Arterial blood pressure
   (c) Blood haemoglobin concentration
   (d) Blood volume

Peripheral limitations

3. *Peripheral circulation*
   (a) Regional distribution of blood flow
   (b) Muscle blood flow
   (c) Muscle capillary density

   (d) Oxygen diffusion
   (e) Affinity of haemoglobin for oxygen

4. *Muscle metabolism*
   (a) Mitochondrial density
   (b) Oxidative enzyme activities
   (c) Energy stores and substrate availability
   (d) Muscle mass
   (e) Fibre type composition

atmosphere to the site of utilization in the mitochondria of the exercising muscles is essential. In the absence of pulmonary disease, the first stage of this process, the transfer of oxygen from the atmosphere to the blood passing through the pulmonary capillaries, is not usually a limiting factor in man, and lung-function tests on élite marathon runners do not distinguish them from the general healthy population. In animal athletes that possess a relatively greater muscle mass: body mass ratio, such as the thoroughbred horse, respiratory function can be a limiting factor, and, as a consequence, such animals show a significant degree of arterial hypoxemia during very intense exercise. There is some evidence that this also occurs in élite human endurance athletes who possess a very high $\dot{V}O_2$max. Individuals with a high $\dot{V}O_2$max have been shown to possess a high maximum cardiac output. Just as tissue oxygen consumption can be described by the Fick equation described above, whole-body oxygen consumption can similarly be expressed thus:

$$\dot{V}O_2 \text{ of whole body} = \text{Cardiac output} \times (C_aO_2 - C_vO_2).$$

In this equation, the term C_vO_2 represents the oxygen content of mixed venous blood, since veins draining different tissues will have different oxygen contents. The difference in oxygen content between arterial and mixed venous blood is sometimes referred to as 'mean whole-body oxygen extraction'. Maximum heart rate does not appear to be different in endurance athletes, but such individuals do exhibit a higher than normal stroke volume, as a consequence of increased heart size. Well-trained endurance athletes also display an increased extraction of oxygen from the blood; these and other adaptations are discussed in more detail in Chapter 8. The oxygen-carrying capacity of the blood, in terms of ml

O_2 per litre of blood, is certainly not greater in well-trained individuals; if anything it is usually less because of a lower haemoglobin concentration, although total blood volume is greater than in sedentary controls. Experiments in which red cells were re-infused back into well-trained subjects showed that this procedure can temporarily increase $\dot{V}O_2$max, suggesting that the principal limitation to $\dot{V}O_2$max in the healthy, fit individual is the delivery of oxygen to the working muscle. Increasing the mass of active muscle by adding arm-crank activity to cycle ergometry when subjects were at, or close to, their $\dot{V}O_2$max did not elicit a further increase in oxygen consumption, adding further support to the notion of a central cardiovascular limitation to $\dot{V}O_2$max. Based on *in vitro* measurements of muscle oxidative capacity, Saltin (1985) has estimated that the total-body muscle oxidative capacity, when fully activated, far exceeds the capacity of the circulation to deliver oxygen to it.

Many studies have reported falls in both $\dot{V}O_2$max and maximum heart rate (and, therefore, maximum cardiac output) with increasing age, and it is known that there is a close relationship between changes in stroke volume and changes in $\dot{V}O_2$max in both longitudinal training and detraining studies.

1.12 Key points

1. Skeletal muscle cells are long, striated multinucleated fibres. Skeletal muscles are attached to the bones, and can be controlled voluntarily, allowing movement and maintenance of posture.

2. Myofibrils are the contractile elements, composed of chains of sarcomeres containing thin (actin) and thick (myosin) filaments arranged in a regular array. The heads of the myosin molecules form crossbridges that bind reversibly to the actin filaments, causing the filaments to slide over each other toward the centres of the sarcomeres.

3. Regulation of skeletal muscle contraction involves the release of calcium from the sarcoplasmic reticulum following transmission of an action potential along the sarcolemma. Calcium initiates crossbridge activity and sliding of the filaments. Crossbridge activity ends when calcium ions are pumped back into the sarcoplasmic reticulum.

4. There are three types of muscle fibres, classified according to their contractile speed and metabolic characteristics, i.e. Type I (slow-twitch oxidative), Type IIa (fast-twitch oxidative), and Type IIb (fast-twitch glycolytic). Most muscles contain a mixture of fibre types.

5. The energy source for muscle contraction is ATP, which is continuously regenerated during exercise from phosphocreatine, the anaerobic metabolism of glycogen or glucose, or the aerobic metabolism of acetyl-CoA derived principally from the breakdown of carbohydrate or lipid.

6. The TCA cycle and oxidative phosphorylation occur in the mitochondria. In the aerobic resynthesis of ATP, the primary role of oxygen is to act as the

final electron acceptor in the electron transport chain and to combine with hydrogen to form water.

7. Several factors influence the type of substrate used to fuel muscular work. These include: substrate availability; diet; intensity and duration of exercise; training status; hormones; prior exercise; and environmental conditions.

8. During exercise, cardiac output and the ventilation rate increase in relation to exercise intensity, and the increased blood flow is directed towards the active musculature. During maximal exercise, the working muscles extract most of the oxygen delivered to them.

9. The principal limitation to maximal oxygen uptake in healthy humans is probably the maximum cardiac output that can be achieved. Thus, the limitation is related to the ability of the cardiovascular system to deliver oxygen to the working muscles, not the ability of the muscles to extract the oxygen from the blood.

Further reading

Astrand, P. -O. and Rodahl, K. (1986). *Textbook of work physiology* (3rd edn). McGraw-Hill, New York.

Brooks, G. A. and Fahey, T. D. (1984). *Exercise physiology: human bioenergetics and its applications*. John Wiley, New York.

Fox, E. L., Bowers, R. W., and Foss, M. L. (1993). *The physiological basis for exercise and sport*. W. C. Brown, Dubuque, IA.

Marieb, E. N. (1993). *Human anatomy and physiology* (2nd edn). Benjamin Cummings, Redwood City, LA.

Powers, S. K. and Howley, E. T. (1990). *Exercise physiology. Theory and application to fitness and performance*. W. C. Brown, Dubuque, IA.

Stryer, L. (1988). *Biochemistry* (2nd edn). W. H. Freeman, San Francisco, CA.

References

Galbo, H. (1983). *Hormonal and metabolic adaptation to exercise*. Georg Thieme Verlag, New York.

Grimby, and Saltin, B. (1983). The ageing muscle. *Clin. Physiol.*, **3**, 209–81.

Komi, G. V. and Karlsson, J. (1978). Skeletal muscle fibre types, enzyme activities and physical performance in young males and females. *Acta Physiol. Scand.*, **103**, 210–18.

Poliner, L. R. (1980). Left ventricular performance in normal subjects: a comparison of the responses to exercise in upright and supine positions. *Circulation*, **62**, 528.

Saltin, B. (1985). Physiological adaptation to physical conditioning. *Acta Med. Scand.*, Suppl. 711, 11–24.

2
Purine nucleotides and phosphocreatine

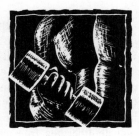

2.1 Free energy

According to the second law of thermodynamics, during any biochemical reaction a certain amount of energy will be transformed into a random disordered form which is unavailable to do work (*entropy*). In addition, *free energy* and *heat energy* (*enthalpy*) will also become available. The former, which is usually signified by the symbol G, can be used to do work at a constant temperature and pressure. It is normally the case that energy transformation in skeletal muscle takes place at a constant temperature and pressure and, therefore, the changes in free energy, enthalpy, and entropy can be described by the following equation:

$$\Delta G = \Delta H - T\,\Delta S;$$

↗ heat

where ΔG is the change in free energy, ΔH is the change in enthalpy, T is the absolute temperature (°K) and ΔS is the change in entropy. Note that it is the changes in free energy, enthalpy, and entropy that are used rather than their absolute quantities.

Every reaction has a characteristic ΔG. Furthermore, it can be seen from the above equation that it is possible to calculate the free energy of any biochemical reaction, assuming standard conditions of temperature (298 °K), pressure (101 kPa), and pH (7.0).

The simplest definition of ΔG for a biochemical reaction is the difference in free energy content between the reactants and the products under standard conditions. For example, assuming the following reaction:

$$A + B \leftrightarrow C + D.$$

The ΔG will be less than zero when the sum of the free energy contents of C and D is less than that of A and B. In this situation, the reaction will tend to occur spontaneously in a rightward direction. If the ΔG is positive the reaction cannot occur spontaneously in this direction and will only occur if energy is added to the system; however, the reaction will occur spontaneously in the opposite direction without the addition of energy. If the ΔG is zero the reaction will proceed in neither direction and will be said to be in a state of equilibrium.

↗ why temp? rise with exercise

2.2 Adenosine triphosphate (ATP) and phosphocreatine (PCr)

Free energy released during the combustion of carbohydrates and lipids can be stored in the compound ATP, hence the terms 'high-energy phosphate' or 'phosphagen', which are commonly used to describe this compound. ATP is the only form of chemical energy that can be converted into other forms of energy used by living cells. For example, the hydrolysis of ATP to ADP and P_i by skeletal muscle liberates free energy enabling force generation to occur. Reactions involving the breakdown of the phosphate bonds and the liberation of P_i are catalysed by enzymes called kinases. In the case of ATP breakdown, these are commonly abbreviated to ATPases. Furthermore, the cellular concentrations of ATP, ADP, and P_i are such that the ΔG of the adenylate kinase reactions (also known as the myokinase reactions) depicted below are large and negative, thereby enabling enough chemical energy to be converted into mechanical work to produce force or movement.

$$ATP \rightarrow ADP + P_i \text{ and } ATP \rightarrow AMP + 2P_i.$$

It has been shown that muscles can perform up to 24 kJ of work for each mole of ATP degraded. It follows, therefore, that the ΔG for ATP hydrolysis must be greater than 24 kJ mole^{-1}. It is also worth noting that the component parts of the adenylate kinase reaction are interconvertible without any net change in ΔG:

$$ATP \rightarrow AMP \leftrightarrow ADP + ADP.$$

The structure of ATP is shown in Fig. 2.1. It is a nucleotide consisting of the purine base adenine, the five-carbon sugar ribose, and a triphosphate unit.

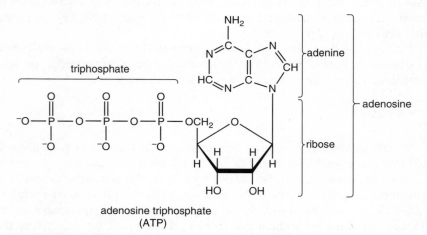

adenosine triphosphate
(ATP)

Fig. 2.1 Adenosine triphosphate consists of an adenine, a ribose sugar, and a triphosphate unit.

Generally, the most metabolically active form of ATP is the magnesium salt and the most interesting part of the compound, in terms of exercise metabolism, is the triphosphate unit. The sequential hydrolysis of the two terminal phosphate bonds in the adenylate kinase reactions releases a substantial amount of free energy that is used to drive a myriad of energy-requiring reactions and processes, including muscle force generation, the pumping of ions across membranes, and all reactions involved in the synthesis of complex compounds:

$$ATP + H_2O \rightarrow ADP + P_i + H^+ : \Delta G = -31 \text{ kJ mole}^{-1};$$

$$ADP + H_2O \rightarrow AMP + P_i + H^+ : \Delta G = -31 \text{ kJ mole}^{-1}.$$

It should be noted that there is nothing particularly special about the phosphate bonds in the above reactions. Their importance lies in that they release free energy when hydrolysed.

Due to its unique role in energy production, ATP has been termed the energy currency of the cell. However, unlike money, ATP cannot be accumulated in large amounts and the intramuscular ATP store is limited to 24 mmol kg dry material^{-1} (dm; Fig. 2.2). Indeed, given that changes in the cellular concentrations of ATP, ADP, and AMP are involved in the regulation of many metabolic processes (see discussion of cellular energy charge below), it would be unwise to simply increase the cellular store of ATP. During maximal exercise, there is sufficient ATP present to fuel about 2 s of contraction. However, the muscle ATP store never becomes completely depleted because it is normally efficiently resynthesized from ADP and AMP at the same rate at which it is

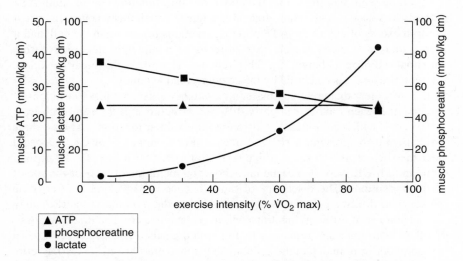

Fig. 2.2 Muscle ATP, phosphocreatine, and lactate concentrations at different exercise intensities in man. Muscle biopsy samples were obtained following 3 min of cycling exercise at each work rate.

degraded. During submaximal, steady-state exercise this is achieved by mito-chondrial oxidation of carbohydrates and lipids (see Chapter 7). However, during the rest to steady-state transition period at the onset of submaximal exer-cise this is achieved principally by anaerobic ATP resynthesis. It has been demonstrated that there is a clear relationship between the rates of PCr hydro-lysis, lactate production, and exercise intensity at the onset of submaximal exer-cise (Fig. 2.2). As referred to in Chapter 7, it is unclear whether these responses occur because of a lag in oxygen delivery and/or inertia in the activation of mitochondrial ATP resynthesis (TCA cycle and oxidative phosphorylation) at the onset of contraction. During brief maximal exercise, the rate of ATP demand far exceeds the capacity of mitochondrial ATP resynthesis and, therefore, anaer-obic metabolism becomes the dominant contributor to ATP resynthesis (see Chapter 6). In physiological terms, this contribution from anaerobic metabolism to ATP resynthesis, whether at the onset of submaximal exercise or during high-intensity exercise, appears as the oxygen deficit.

Phosphocreatine is restricted to the cytoplasm of the muscle cell where it is present at a concentration of about 75 mmol kg dm^{-1} (Fig. 2.2). The rapid de-gradation of PCr at the onset of submaximal exercise and during high-intensity exercise occurs because it has a higher phosphate-group transfer potential than ATP. This means that the free energy of PCr hydrolysis ($-$ 43 kJ mole^{-1}) is greater than that of ATP ($-$ 31 kJ mole^{-1}), resulting in a greater likelihood for free energy transfer to occur from PCr to ADP to re-form ATP:

$$ADP + PCr + H^+ \rightarrow ATP + Cr.$$

It can be seen, therefore, that the above reaction functions to maintain ATP homeostasis during contraction. Indeed, the rate at which this reaction can occur is far in excess of any of the ATP utilizing reactions occurring in the cell, and it is not unusual for the muscle PCr store to be completely degraded during maximal exercise (Chapter 6). This reaction is termed the creatine kinase reaction because it is catalysed by the enzyme creatine kinase.

It is now clear that creatine kinase has a number of isoenzymes (variations of the enzyme, each having a slightly different structure but the same substrate specificity), which are located at different intracellular locations. At least three are known to be present in skeletal muscle. For example, MM-CK is located near the sites of muscle crossbridge formation (i.e. near a site of ATP utiliza-tion) and Mi-CK is located at the mitochondrial membrane (i.e. near the site of ATP production). The discovery of the existence of isoenzymes of creatine kinase with discrete cellular locations has led to the hypothesis that PCr may have a number of different functions within skeletal muscle. The first, and possi-bly the most important, relates to its function described above, i.e. acting as a temporal buffer to maintain the cellular ATP concentration and ATP:ADP ratio. A second function, which is currently the subject of much debate, is that PCr may act as a spatial energy buffer, i.e. an energy transport system between the site of ATP production (the mitochondria) and the sites of ATP utilization (e.g.

the myofibrils). This suggested function has resulted in the use of the phrase 'the PCr shuttle'. Those researchers in favour of its existence have gone on to suggest that the primary role for PCr in Type I muscle fibres may be to operate as a spatial buffer, which contrasts with its suggested principal role in Type II fibres as a temporal energy buffer. The 10–20 mmol kg dm^{-1} higher concentration of PCr found in Type II fibres supports this suggestion. A third suggested function for PCr is its functional coupling with several other cellular reactions, which facilitates the integration of energy metabolism during muscle contraction. For example, it is clear from the reactions described above that the adenylate kinase reaction will result in the generation of H$^+$ and the creatine kinase reaction will result in the sequestering of H$^+$; it is the functional coupling of these two reactions which prevents the rapid acidification of the cell at the onset of contraction. Similarly, the rapid liberation of P$_i$ by PCr hydrolysis during contraction plays an integral part in the activation of glycogen phosphorylase at the onset of exercise, thereby ensuring that energy production is maintained.

The creatine kinase reaction is an equilibrium reaction (as is the adenylate kinase reaction) and is therefore reversible. This will occur following exercise when the energy charge of the cell is increased (see discussion of energy charge below) and sufficient free energy is available to rephosphorylate creatine (Cr):

$$ATP + Cr \rightarrow ADP + PCr + H^+.$$

In general, the resynthesis of PCr following complete degradation follows an exponential curve and the half-time for resynthesis (the time to resynthesize 50% of the resting store) is often quoted as 30 s (Fig. 2.3). In reality, however, there appears to be an enormous variation in the time-course of resynthesis depending on the type of exercise performed and the duration and number of exercise bouts completed. Factors known to influence the rate of PCr resynthesis during recovery from exercise are the cellular concentrations of ATP, ADP, and Cr, which is not surprising given the equilibrium nature of the creatine kinase reaction (the effect of muscle Cr availability on PCr resynthesis following Cr ingestion is discussed in Chapter 6). In addition, the H$^+$ is known to be a potent inhibitor of creatine kinase. Therefore, in practice a low muscle pH, a low oxygen tension, and/or a reduction in muscle blood flow will severely impair PCr resynthesis following exercise. Indeed, muscle ischaemia is often used as a tool in metabolic research to 'arrest' PCr resynthesis following muscle contraction, thereby providing sufficient time to enable relevant biochemical and physiological measurements to be made (Fig. 2.3).

It is now clear that there are differences in the rates of PCr resynthesis between muscle fibre types following exercise-induced PCr depletion. This point will be discussed in more detail in Chapter 6. Briefly, it seems that the rate of PCr resynthesis is significantly lower in Type II muscle fibres during the initial minutes of recovery (possibly due to a greater lactic acidosis in this fibre type),

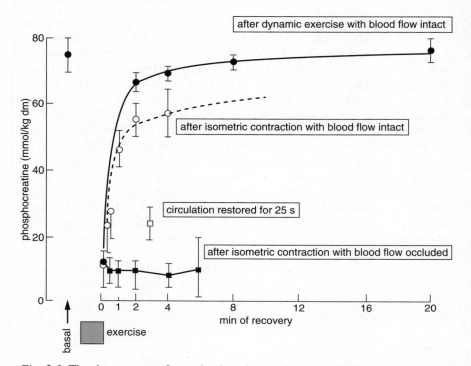

Fig. 2.3 The time course of muscle phosphocreatine resynthesis during recovery from exhaustive high-intensity cycling exercise with muscle blood flow intact (filled circles). The same measurements are also depicted following exhaustive isometric contraction with blood flow intact (open circles), blood flow occluded (filled squares), and after 25 s following restoration of blood flow (open square). (From Harris *et al.* 1976.)

which has been shown to have an adverse effect on energy production and exercise performance during a subsequent bout of exercise. Following these initial few minutes though, PCr resynthesis is accelerated in Type II muscle fibres, such that after 15 min of recovery the concentration of PCr is actually greater than that observed at rest. The mechanism responsible for this PCr overshoot in Type II fibres is currently unknown.

2.3 The free energy charge and the adenylate pool

The concentrations of ATP, ADP, and AMP can be used to calculate the energy charge of the cell. This concept was proposed by Atkinson (1977; and see Further reading) and it is a measure of the extent to which the total adenine nucleotide pool of the cell (ATP, ADP, and AMP) is phosphorylated. It is described by the following equation:

$$\text{Energy charge} = \frac{[ATP] + 0.5[ADP]}{[ATP] + [ADP] + [AMP]}.$$

The energy charge is a good indicator of the energy status of the cell (i.e. its capacity to do work). For example, the energy charge of the cell will be 1.0 when the whole of the adenine nucleotide pool is in the form of ATP, and under these conditions the cell will have a maximum free-energy charge. Conversely, the energy charge will be zero when ATP has been completely hydrolysed to AMP. This latter scenario should only be viewed as a theoretical example, since the concentration of ATP in human skeletal muscle will not decline by more than 60%, even during maximal exercise with blood flow completely occluded. Under normal resting conditions, the energy charge of skeletal muscle is in the region of 0.90–0.95. However, this has been shown to decline to less than 0.9 in some disease states (e.g. sepsis), with a value of less than 0.82 being indicative of irreversible cellular damage.

The rate of ATP resynthesis during exercise is known to be regulated by the energy charge of the muscle cell. For example, the decrease in the energy charge at the onset of contraction, i.e. the momentary decline in ATP and increases in ADP and AMP, accelerates both anaerobic and oxidative ATP resynthesis, with the net effect of increasing the rate of energy supply to match the increased demand. If the energy charge continues to decline ATP degradation will be inhibited, i.e. the muscle will fatigue and work output will fall. The relationships between the energy charge and the rates of ATP degradation and resynthesis during exercise are depicted in Fig. 2.4. The rate of ATP production during contraction will match that of utilization where the two lines intersect. It can be seen that if the energy charge rises or falls from this steady state then ATP, ADP, and AMP will act as allosteric activators or inhibitors of the enzymatic reactions involved in PCr, carbohydrate, and fat degradation and utilization. For example, as already mentioned, creatine kinase, the enzyme responsible for the rapid rephosphorylation of ATP at the initiation of contraction, is rapidly activated by an increase in cytoplasmic ADP concentration (a decrease in the energy charge) and is inhibited by an increase in cellular ATP concentration (an increase in the energy charge). Similarly, glycogen phosphorylase, the enzyme which catalyses the conversion of glycogen to glucose 1-phosphate, is activated by increases in AMP and P_i and is inhibited by an increase in ATP concentration.

A word of caution, however: because the energy charge is calculated from the total tissue contents of adenine nucleotides measured in muscle, it does not take into account the proportion of adenine nucleotides that are unavailable to influence metabolic control. For example, the metabolically active (free) forms of ADP and AMP are considered to be considerably lower than their respective total cellular concentrations (free + bound). It is clear, therefore, that changes in the free forms of these compounds will not always be reflected in a change in

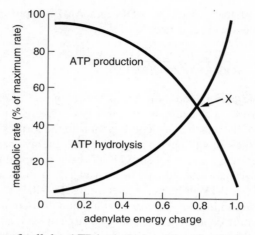

Fig. 2.4 The rates of cellular ATP hydrolysis and production as a function of the cellular energy charge. At the point of intersection (x), the rate of ATP production matches the rate of ATP hydrolysis and the cell is in a steady state of energy turnover.

the energy charge of the cell as a whole. More recently, magnetic resonance spectroscopy has been used to measure the concentrations of bound and free phosphates, thereby attempting to avoid this problem. With this technique has come the convention of using the ratios of ATP to ADP and PCr to ATP to indicate the free-energy status of the cell.

It is important to differentiate between the energy charge and the total adenylate pool of muscle (the sum of cellular ATP, ADP, and AMP concentrations). It is known that the total adenylate pool can decline rapidly if the AMP concentration of the cell begins to rise during muscle force generation. This decline occurs principally via deamination of AMP to inosine monophosphate (IMP) but also by the dephosphorylation of AMP to adenosine (see below). The loss of AMP may initially appear counterproductive because of the reduction in the total adenylate pool. However, it should be noted that the deamination of AMP to IMP only occurs under low-energy charge conditions and, by preventing excessive accumulation of ADP and AMP, enables the adenylate kinase reactions to continue, resulting in an increase in the energy charge and continuing contraction. Furthermore, it is has been proposed that the free energy of ATP hydrolysis will decrease when ADP and P_i accumulate, which could further impair contraction. For these reasons, it has been suggested that adenine nucleotide loss is important to muscle function during conditions of metabolic crisis; for example during maximal exercise and in the later stages of prolonged submaximal exercise when glycogen stores become depleted.

2.4 Skeletal muscle adenine nucleotide loss

As Fig. 2.5 indicates, skeletal muscle adenine nucleotide loss can occur in two ways during exercise. First, there is the deamination of AMP to IMP and ammonia, catalysed by AMP-deaminase. Second, there is the dephosphorylation of AMP to adenosine, catalysed by 5-nucleotidase. IMP and adenosine can be further degraded to inosine and hypoxanthine. Muscle does not possess the enzymes required to convert hypoxanthine to inosine and, therefore, once formed hypoxanthine tends to leave muscle and is eventually converted to uric acid in the liver, which is then excreted via the kidneys. Alternatively, IMP can be converted to adenylosuccinate and eventually back to AMP. The deamination of AMP to IMP and the subsequent reamination of IMP constitutes the purine . nucleotide cycle which will be discussed in more detail later.

As indicated previously, it is suggested that adenine nucleotide loss occurs during intense muscle contraction in an attempt to enable the adenylate kinase reactions to continue and thereby maintain a high energy charge. This loss has

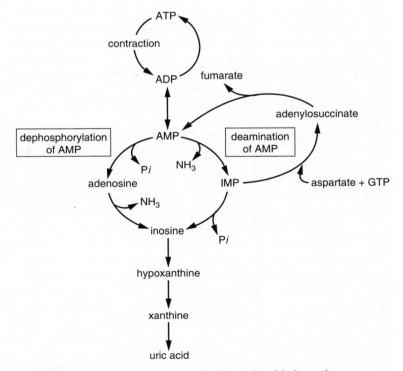

Fig. 2.5 Pathways of skeletal muscle adenine nucleotide loss via dephosphorylation and deamination.

been shown to be matched by stoichiometric increases in IMP and ammonia concentrations (Fig. 2.5). It is for this reason that the appearances of ammonia and hypoxanthine in plasma are often used as non-invasive indicators of muscle adenine nucleotide loss during exercise.

It is clear from the literature that the predominant pathway for adenine nucleotide loss during exercise differs between muscle fibre types and species. For example, the deamination of AMP to IMP is the dominant pathway in fast-contracting muscle (containing predominantly Type II fibres) in the *rat*. In slow-contracting *rat* muscle (containing predominantly Type I fibres), adenine nucleotide loss does not usually occur unless an extreme metabolic crisis occurs (e.g. muscle ischaemia). However, even under these extreme conditions, adenine nucleotide loss will not occur via deamination, but rather by dephosphorylation to adenosine or, perhaps, a yet to be elucidated pathway. By way of contrast, deamination of AMP to IMP also occurs in Type I *human* muscle fibres, albeit at a much lesser extent than that observed in human Type II muscle fibres. These findings fit with the approximately 4-fold lower activity of AMP deaminase measured in Type I human muscle fibres compared with Type II human fibres and with the comparatively higher activity compared with rat slow fibres. It is unclear why the route and rate of adenine nucleotide loss during exercise differs between fibre types. One explanation offered is that because the accumulation of IMP and ammonia has been implicated with the activation of glycogen phosphorylase and phosphofructokinase, the comparatively greater accumulation of both in fast-contracting muscle may be involved in the rapid activation of glycogenolysis and glycolysis in this type of muscle during intense contraction. However, the observed activation of glycogenolysis and glycolysis before significant amounts of IMP and ammonia have accumulated goes against this suggestion.

An alternative explanation for the differences in adenine nucleotide loss between fibre types, is that the formation of adenosine by slow-contracting muscle facilitates vasodilatation and thereby promotes blood flow to these oxygen-dependent fibres. This hypothesis is supported by the high vasoactive nature of adenosine. It should be stressed, however, that there is a lack of definitive experimental data to support any of the above interpretations. This aside, it is clear from the literature that the principal pathway of adenine nucleotide loss in *human* skeletal muscle is via the deamination of AMP to IMP and ammonia. Finally, it is important to recognize that the binding of AMP deaminase to myosin is vital to the activation of the enzyme and must occur before deamination of AMP can take place. Thus, at rest, the enzyme is inactive and appears to be free in the cytosol. However, at the onset of high force generation a large proportion of the enzyme becomes bound to myosin. It would appear that the high energy demand of muscle force generation rather than the crossbridge mechanism *per se* is important to this binding process. For example, low force generation is known to have no influence on AMP deaminase binding or IMP formation.

2.5 The purine nucleotide cycle

The reactions that make up the purine nucleotide cycle are depicted in Fig. 2.6. These three reactions are confined to the muscle cytosol and are catalysed by AMP deaminase, adenylosuccinate synthetase, and adenylosuccinate lyase. The cycle can be conveniently divided into deamination (catalysed by AMP deaminase) and reamination (catalysed by adenylosuccinate synthetase and adenylosuccinate lyase) pathways. As discussed in some detail above, the deamination pathway of the purine nucleotide cycle is important to the regulation of adenine nucleotide metabolism in muscle. However, the purine nucleotide cycle has a number of other functions which should be identified.

2.5.1 Deamination in the purine nucleotide cycle

The deamination of AMP to IMP and ammonia has been discussed previously in relation to this pathway, being the principal mechanism of adenine nucleotide loss in human skeletal muscle during exercise. It has been known for several decades that contracting muscle produces IMP and ammonia from the deamination of AMP, that this reaction is irreversible, and that it is catalysed by AMP

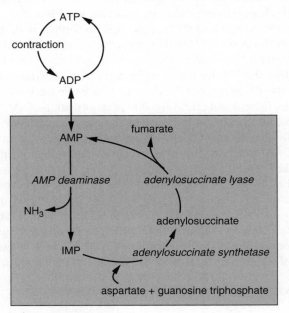

purine nucleotide cycle

Fig. 2.6 The purine nucleotide cycle (in box).

deaminase (Fig. 2.6). As might be predicted from the previous discussion of cellular energy charge, AMP, ADP, ATP, and P_i are important regulators of AMP deaminase activation. The activity of the enzyme is also pH-dependent, but AMP deaminase binding to myosin can still occur in the absence of acidosis. Thus, the metabolic conditions in resting muscle (high energy charge and pH 7.0) result in the inactivation of the enzyme. However, the decrease in energy charge during intense exercise, together with the exercise-induced acidosis (due to lactic acid production), result in the activation of the enzyme and the formation of IMP and ammonia. It should be noted, however, that the increase in ADP and AMP can act independently of pH to activate AMP deaminase. For example, it has been demonstrated that the depletion of muscle glycogen stores during prolonged exercise, which produces increases in ADP and AMP, but reduces lactic acid production, results in AMP deaminase activation. Similarly, the muscle of patients with McArdle's disease, which lacks glycogen phosphorylase, has been shown to produce IMP and ammonia, despite the absence of lactic acid formation. Conversely, the correlation between blood and muscle lactate accumulation and ammonia and hypoxanthine accumulation during incremental exercise in healthy individuals is good evidence that AMP deaminase is activated by acidosis. Indeed, AMP deaminase activity in slow, rat skeletal muscle has been shown to be increased only when muscle pH declines below 6.6.

Several roles for the deamination pathway of the purine nucleotide cycle have been proposed. Probably the most important is its role in the maintenance of the cellular energy charge during exercise. This role has been discussed in some detail already and, therefore, will be addressed no further, with the exception, however, that the formation of IMP during contraction could, in addition to maintaining energy status by reducing the adenylate pool, also provide an energetically efficient mechanism for the re-expansion of the adenylate pool following exercise. Because the process of *de novo* (new) adenine nucleotide synthesis is energetically inefficient and relatively slow, the formation of IMP represents a more favourable mechanism for replenishing the adenine nucleotide pool. The literature indicates that the adenylate pool is normally restored within 1 h of recovery from maximal exercise. However, recent evidence demonstrates that this process can take longer (more than 3 days) following a 1–6-week period of high-intensity training. This delay is most likely to be due to the degradation of IMP to hypoxanthine, thereby necessitating *de novo* purine synthesis. Interestingly, however, high-intensity training did appear to result in an adaptation whereby less adenine nucleotide loss occurred during exercise following training.

Ammonia formed during the deamination of AMP has been suggested to be of importance in the buffering of H^+ produced during intense exercise:

$$NH_3 + H^+ \rightarrow NH_4^+.$$

However, given that the magnitude of H^+ formation during exercise is likely to be at least 50-fold greater than that of ammonia this explanation appears to be quantitatively unimportant.

As briefly mentioned earlier, IMP and ammonia accumulation during exercise has been associated with the regulation of carbohydrate utilization. IMP has been implicated with the activation of glycogen phosphorylase b and thereby glycogenolysis during contraction. However, this role for IMP seems unlikely, given that the extent of IMP accumulation observed during exercise would be insufficient to sustain the high rates of glycogenolysis observed during intense exercise. More recent evidence points to AMP being a more potent regulator of glycogenolysis during exercise. The ammonium ion (NH_4^+) has been shown to activate phosphofructokinase *in vitro* and therefore its accumulation during exercise has been implicated with the regulation of glycolysis. However, as stated previously, the fact that glycogenolysis and glycolysis can be accelerated before IMP and ammonium accumulation occurs points to them playing only a minor (if any) role in the control of carbohydrate degradation.

2.5.2 Reamination in the purine nucleotide cycle

Fig. 2.6 demonstrates that the reamination pathway of the purine nucleotide cycle is catalysed by adenylosuccinate synthetase and adenylosuccinate lyase. Adenylosuccinate synthetase catalyses the formation of adenylosuccinate from IMP, aspartate, and guanosine triphosphate. It is the rate-limiting step in the purine nucleotide cycle. Adenylosuccinate lyase catalyses the formation of AMP and fumarate from adenylosuccinate.

It would appear that the role of reamination in the purine nucleotide cycle differs depending on the metabolic conditions prevailing. For example, during intense muscle contraction it is clear that deamination dominates and that re-amination would be counterproductive under such conditions. Indeed, there is little (if any) evidence to demonstrate that reamination occurs during high muscle force generation. However, during prolonged low/moderate-intensity exercise it would appear that the purine nucleotide cycle may be operative. It would seem, however, that the reamination pathway may be occurring in non-activated fibres during prolonged exercise; i.e. implying that deamination and reamination do not occur concomitantly. This aside, it can be seen from Fig. 2.6 that one complete turn of the cycle will result in the utilization of aspartate and the formation of fumarate and ammonia, without any net change in AMP and IMP concentrations. As fumarate is an intermediate of the tricarboxylic acid (TCA) cycle, it has been suggested that the purine nucleotide cycle may contribute to the expansion of the TCA cycle intermediates (anaplerosis) which occurs at the onset of exercise. Thus, the purine nucleotide cycle may enhance mitochondrial respiration by increasing the rates of acetyl-CoA oxidation and NADH formation and thereby may be at least partly responsible for maintaining muscle function during exercise. A word of caution, however: the observed expansion of TCA cycle intermediates during high-intensity exercise, in the absence of reamination, suggests that the anaplerotic role of the purine nucleotide cycle is of only minor importance. Indeed, recent evidence points to carbohydrate availability being the principal determinant of TCA cycle intermediate availability. Furthermore, there is no evidence to show that a decline in mitochondrial respiration or NADH concentration occurs during prolonged exercise suggesting, therefore, that the availability of TCA cycle intermediates does not limit mitochondrial respiration.

2.5.3 Fatigue

The close association between muscle adenine nucleotide loss and fatigue development during short-lasting intense exercise and prolonged submaximal exercise points to AMP deamination being implicated with fatigue development. However, it is likely that this association merely reflects the failure of energy delivery via PCr hydrolysis, glycolysis, and oxidative phosphorylation to meet the demands of muscle force generation (see Chapters 6 and 7), resulting in increases in ADP and AMP (a decrease in the cellular energy charge), the activation of AMP deaminase, and, ultimately, the development of fatigue due to a local lack of ATP and/or accumulation of ADP. Support for this conclusion comes from metabolic disease states (e.g. McArdle's syndrome) where the impairment of energy delivery is paralleled by enhanced rates of adenine nucleotide loss and fatigue development during exercise. Alternatively, however, recent evidence shows that fatigue development in AMP deaminase-deficient patients, who lack the capacity to form IMP, is no different from control subjects. In addition, studies have shown an improvement in high-intensity cycling exercise performance following a high-intensity training programme, despite a 20% decrease in the adenine nucleotide pool. Taken together, these findings point to muscle fatigue development being a multifactorial process not necessarily related to muscle energy metabolism.

2.6 Key points

1. During any biochemical reaction free energy will be released which can then be used to do work. In muscle, free energy released during the combustion of carbohydrates and lipids can be stored as chemical energy in the form of ATP. Free energy released by the subsequent degradation of ATP in the ATPase reactions can be converted into mechanical energy to produce work (muscle can perform 24 kJ of work for each mole of ATP degraded). ATP is the only compound in living cells that enables this energy conversion to take place.

2. Phosphocreatine is present in the cytosol of muscle at about three times the concentration of ATP. It is generally accepted that the rapid degradation of PCr in the creatine kinase reaction at the onset of muscle force generation occurs because the free energy released can be used to resynthesize ATP, thereby maintaining a high cellular ATP:ADP ratio. However, the discovery of several isoenzymes of creatine kinase, each with defined cellular locations, has led to the hypothesis that PCr may have a number of different functions within skeletal muscle.

3. The creatine kinase reaction is reversible and occurs following exercise when sufficient energy is available to rephosphorylate Cr. The resynthesis of PCr follows an exponential curve, but the time-course of resynthesis is dependent on a number of factors.

4. The sum of cellular ATP, ADP, and AMP concentrations is termed the total adenine nucleotide pool. The extent to which the total adenine nucleotide pool is phosphorylated is known as the energy charge of the cell, and it is a good indicator of the energy status of the cell. The rate at which ATP is resynthesized during exercise is known to be regulated by the energy charge of the muscle cell. For example, the decline in cellular concentration of ATP at the onset of muscle force generation and parallel increases in ADP and AMP concentrations (i.e. a decline in the energy charge) will directly stimulate anaerobic and oxidative ATP resynthesis.

5. The total adenine nucleotide pool of the cell will decline if the AMP concentration of the cell begins to rise during exercise. The loss of adenine nucleotides is potentially detrimental because it will reduce the availability of adenine nucleotides for phosphorylation. However, this adverse effect is outweighed in the short term by the stimulatory effect that the reduction in the cellular ADP and AMP concentrations has on the adenylate kinase reactions, resulting in an increase in the energy charge and continued force generation.

6. Skeletal muscle adenine nucleotide loss occurs, first, by the deamination of AMP to IMP and ammonia and, second, by the dephosphorylation of AMP to adenosine. Both IMP and adenosine can be further degraded by the liver to inosine and then hypoxanthine, which then leaves muscle and is degraded by the liver and excreted by the kidneys. The predominant pathway for adenine nucleotide loss in man is via the deamination of AMP to IMP and ammonia; however, substantial variation is known to exist between muscle fibre types and animal species.

7. An alternative fate for IMP is that it can be used to resynthesize AMP. The deamination of AMP to IMP and subsequent reamination of IMP forms the purine nucleotide cycle. Several important roles have been proposed for the purine nucleotide cycle in muscle energy metabolism.

8. It has been suggested that the close association between muscle adenine nucleotide loss and the development of fatigue during short-lasting intense exercise and prolonged submaximal exercise points to AMP deamination being implicated with fatigue development. However, it is more likely that this association is more a reflection of energy delivery failing to meet the energy demands of the exercise and that fatigue will ultimately be due to a number of factors, including a local cellular depletion of ATP and/or an accumulation of ADP.

Further reading

Aragon, J. J., Tornheim, K., Goodman, M. N., and Lowenstein, J. M. (1981). Replenishment of citric cycle intermediates by the purine nucleotide cycle in rat skeletal muscle. *Curr. Top. Cell Regul.*, **18**, 131–49.

Broberg, S. and Sahlin, K. (1989). Adenine nucleotide degradation in human skeletal muscle during prolonged exercise. *J. Appl. Physiol.*, **67**, 116–22.

Flanagan, W. F., Holmes, E. W., Sabina, R. L., and Swain, J. L. (1986). Importance of purine nucleotide cycle to energy production in skeletal muscle. *Am. J. Physiol.*, **251**, C795–C802.

Hellsten, Y., Norman, B., Balsom, P. D., and Sjodin, B. (1993). Decreased resting levels of adenine nucleotides in human skeletal muscle after high-intensity training. *J. Appl. Physiol.*, **74**, 2524–8.

Katz, A., Sahlin, K., and Henriksson, J. (1986). Muscle ammonia metabolism during isometric contraction in humans. *Am. J. Physiol.*, **250**, C834–C840.

Lowenstein, J. M. (1990). The purine nucleotide cycle revised. *Int. J. Sports Med.*, **11**, S37–46.

McPartland, A. and Segal, I. H. (1986). Equilibrium constants, free energy changes and coupled reactions: concepts and misconcepts. *Biochem. Ed.*, **14**, 137–41.

Meyer, R. A. and Terjung, R. L. (1979). Differences in ammonia and adenylate metabolism in contracting fast and slow muscle. *Am. J. Physiol.*, **237**, C111–C118.

Meyer, R. A. and Terjung, R. L. (1980). AMP deamination and IMP reamination in working skeletal muscle. *Am. J. Physiol.*, **239**, C32–C38.

Ren, J.-M. and Hultman, E. (1989). Regulation of glycogenolysis in human skeletal muscle. *J. Appl. Physiol.*, **67**, 2243–8.

Sahlin, K. and Broberg, S. (1990). Adenine nucleotide depletion in human muscle during exercise: causality and significance of AMP deamination. *Int. J. Sports Med.*, **11**, S62–S67.

Sahlin, K., Katz, A., and Broberg, S. (1990). Tricarboxylic cycle intermediates in human muscle during submaximal exercise. *Am. J. Physiol.*, **259**, C834–C841.

Spencer, M. K., Yan, Z., and Katz, A. (1991). Carbohydrate supplementation attenuates IMP accumulation in human muscle during prolonged exercise. *Am. J. Physiol.*, **261**, C71–C76.

Tullson, P. C. and Terjung, R. L. (1991). Adenine nucleotide metabolism in contracting skeletal muscle. *Exerc. Sport. Sci. Rev.*, **19**, 507–37.

References

Atkinson, D. E. (1977). *Cellular energy metabolism and its regulation.* Academic Press, New York.

Harris, R. C., Edwards, R. H. T., Hultman, E. Nordesjo, L.-O., Nylind, B., and Sahlin, K. (1976). The time course of phosphorylcreatine resynthesis during recovery of the quadriceps muscle in man. *Pflugers Arch.*, **376**, 137–42.

3
Carbohydrate metabolism

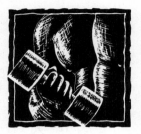

3.1 Role of carbohydrates

It is easy to demonstrate the crucial role played by carbohydrate (CHO) metabolism in supplying energy for physical activity. In high-intensity exercise, the majority of the energy demand is met by energy made available by carbohydrate breakdown. In more moderate-intensity exercise where the duration is longer, performance is commonly limited by the availability of carbohydrate as fuel. The supply of carbohydrate and its metabolism are, therefore, central to the capacity for physical work. Even at rest, failure to maintain the blood glucose concentration, which supplies carbohydrate fuel to the brain and other tissues, results in central nervous dysfunction which can progress to coma and death.

3.2 Carbohydrate supply

Carbohydrate is available to the body from the diet as well as from endogenous reserves, mostly in the form of muscle and liver glycogen. The body also has a limited capacity for the synthesis of glucose from non-carbohydrate precursors. The classification of dietary carbohydrates is described in more detail in Appendix 1, but the important dietary carbohydrates consist of monosaccharides (such as glucose, fructose, galactose) which consist of single sugars, disaccharides (pairs of sugar molecules linked together, such as maltose, lactose), and polysaccharides (such as starch, which consists of long chains of glucose molecules) (Fig. 3.1). The major part of the carbohydrate present in the diet is usually in the form of sucrose and starch, and there are important nutritional and health implications of varying the proportions of these.

Whatever the form in which carbohydrate is consumed, dietary carbohydrate must be digested to its component monosaccharides before absorption can occur: this process involves hydrolysis of the bonds linking the monosaccharides and is illustrated for the degradation of amylopectin (starch) in Fig. 3.2. A limited amount of hydrolysis of carbohydrates occurs in the mouth and in the stomach, but most occurs in the upper part of the small intestine where the pH allows a high activity of the specific enzymes secreted into the intestinal lumen. Some polysaccharides, such as cellulose, in which the component glucose molecules are linked by β-1,4 bonds, are resistant to hydrolysis in the upper part of the human intestine. These pass through the gut largely undigested, although

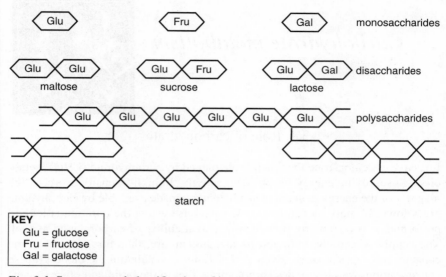

Fig. 3.1 Structure and classification of important dietary carbohydrates and of glycogen, the animal storage form of carbohydrate.

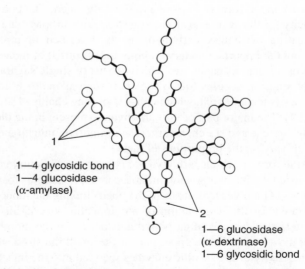

Fig. 3.2 Hydrolysis of the α-1,4 and α-1,6 links in starch during the process of digestion liberates free glucose which is available for absorption. Compare the breakdown of glycogen in muscle (*Fig. 3.4*).

some bacterial fermentation can occur in the lower part of the intestine. The digestive system of ruminants is designed to allow the products of this fermentation process to be available for absorption: these species depend for food on carbohydrates that would be unavailable to the human.

The average western diet contains slightly less than 50% of total energy in the form of carbohydrate: total carbohydrate intake is, therefore, about 300 g per day for the average 70 kg sedentary male consuming 12 MJ (about 3000 kcal) per day. Since the body's carbohydrate reserves are small and remain approximately constant, this must be very close to the daily utilization rate. In a typical 70 kg man, the total-body carbohydrate store amounts to about 300–500 g, mostly in the form of glycogen. The amount consumed each day is therefore, roughly equivalent to the amount of the normal whole-body store. About 80–110 g of CHO is stored in the liver: this acts as a true store, and can be released into the blood for transport to other tissues. The largest CHO store is in skeletal muscle: the typical female, with a smaller tissue mass, will have a smaller CHO store. The muscle glycogen reserve is not readily available to other tissues. The total glucose content of the extracellular fluid amounts to only about 15 g: this should not be regarded as an energy store, as even small decreases in the blood glucose concentration can impair muscle and nerve cell function. Although the muscle glycogen store remains almost unchanged in response to fasting, provided that no strenuous exercise is performed, the liver glycogen content falls rapidly after the postabsorptive period.

The glycogen molecule resembles starch, except that the linkage between the glucose molecules is different (Fig. 3.1). In glycogen, the main glycosidic bond is an α-1,4 carbon bond, with branching points in the molecule resulting from additional α-1,6 bonds after about every 6–10 glucose residues: in starch, there are two polysaccharides present, amylose which consists of long chains of glucose molecules joined by α-1,4 bonds, and amylopectin which has a structure similar to that of glycogen.

3.3 The reactions of anaerobic glycolysis and glycogenolysis

The initial steps in the degradation of the body's carbohydrate stores occur without the involvement of oxygen, and are, therefore, anaerobic processes. The terminology depends on the starting point: degradation of glucose is referred to as glycolysis, whereas glycogenolysis begins with glycogen. Except where glycogen is specifically referred to, the term glycolysis is conveniently used to refer to both processes, which share a common pathway after the first steps. Glycolysis effectively converts a 6-carbon glucose molecule to two 3-carbon molecules: the end-product of aerobic glycolysis is pyruvate, whereas the end-product of anaerobic glycolysis is lactate. In the process of glycolysis, some of the chemical energy liberated by the breaking of bonds is conserved in the form

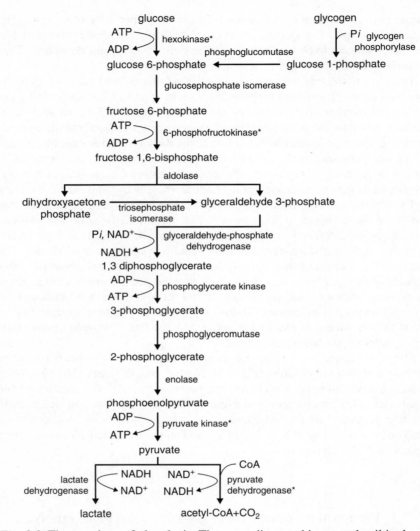

Fig. 3.3 The reactions of glycolysis. These are discussed in more detail in the text.

of ATP. The sequence of reactions which lead to the conversion of glucose or glycogen to pyruvate is shown in Fig. 3.3.

A specific transporter protein (GLUT 4) is involved in the passage of glucose molecules across the cell membrane. Once the glucose molecule is inside the cell, the first step of glycolysis is an irreversible phosphorylation to prevent loss of this valuable nutrient from the cell: glucose is converted to glucose 6-phosphate (G6-P). This step is effectively irreversible, at least as far as muscle is concerned. Liver has a phosphatase enzyme which catalyses the reverse reaction, allowing free glucose to leave the cell and enter the circulation, but this enzyme is absent from muscle. Hexokinase, the enzyme which promotes the phosphorylation of glucose, is intimately linked with the glucose transporter in skeletal muscle, ensuring that the glucose is effectively trapped within the cell. The hexokinase reaction is an energy-consuming reaction, requiring the investment of one molecule of ATP per molecule of glucose. This also ensures a concentration gradient for glucose across the cell membrane down which transport can occur. Hexokinase is inhibited by an accumulation of the reaction product G6P, and during high-intensity exercise, the increasing concentration of G6-P limits the contribution that the blood glucose can make to carbohydrate metabolism in the working muscles.

If glycogen, rather than blood glucose, is the substrate for glycolysis, the first step is to split off a single glucose molecule. This is achieved by the enzyme glycogen phosphorylase, and the products are glucose 1-phosphate (G1-P) and a glycogen molecule that is one glucose residue shorter than the original (Fig. 3.4). The substrates are glycogen and inorganic phosphate, so, unlike the hexokinase reaction, there is no breakdown of ATP in this first reaction. Phosphorylase acts on the α-1,4 carbon bonds at the free ends of the glycogen molecule, but it cannot break the α-1,6 bonds. It stops acting about four glucose units before the branchpoint, and the activity of phosphorylase alone would result in a glycogen molecule consisting of a core with short branches. Further

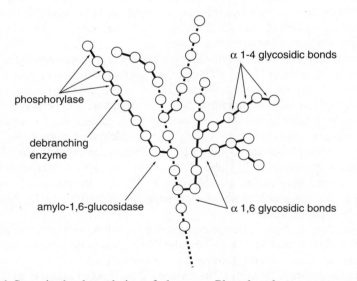

Fig. 3.4 Steps in the degradation of glycogen. Phosphorylase cannot act within about 4-glucose residues of a branchpoint, so further breakdown requires a debranching enzyme. The action of α-1,6-glucosidase at the branchpoints liberates free glucose.

degradation of the glycogen molecule requires the activity of debranching enzyme, which detaches a chain three units long from the end of one branch and re-attaches it by an α-1,4 bond to the end of an adjacent branch. This leaves a single glucose molecule attached by an α-1,6 bond, and this bond is broken by amylo-1,6-glucosidase, releasing free glucose. The free glucose is quickly phosphorylated to G6-P by the action of hexokinase. There is an accumulation of free glucose within the muscle cell only in very high-intensity exercise where glycogenolysis proceeds rapidly: because there are relatively few α-1,6 bonds, no more than about 10% of the glucose residues appear as free glucose.

The enzyme phosphoglucomutase ensures that G1-P formed by the action of phosphorylase on glycogen is rapidly converted to G6-P, which then proceeds down the glycolytic pathway.

Glucose 6-phosphate is converted to fructose 6-phosphate (F6-P) by the enzyme phosphoglucose isomerase: the activity of this enzyme is high, and the reaction can proceed rapidly in either direction. A second phosphorylation step follows, and F6-P is converted to fructose 1,6-diphosphate (FDP). This reaction also requires the phosphate group to be donated from ATP, and is catalysed by phosphofructokinase (PFK). The activity of this complex enzyme is affected by many intracellular factors, and it plays an important role in controlling flux through the pathway. The PFK reaction is the first opportunity for regulation at a point which will affect the metabolism of both glucose and glycogen, and is frequently described as the rate-limiting reaction in glycolysis. In any sequence of metabolic reactions, there can only be one reaction that determines the overall rate at which the sequence can proceed: it can go no faster than the slowest, or rate-limiting, reaction, and PFK is normally the point in glycolysis that determines the rate of the overall reaction.

So far, glycolysis, which is intended to make energy available to the cells, has required the investment of two ATP molecules, with no immediate return.

FDP is split by the enzyme aldolase into two 3-carbon molecules: glyceraldehyde 3-phosphate and dihydroxyacetone phosphate. These two molecules are interconvertible under the influence of triose phosphate isomerase, and further metabolism occurs only through glyceraldehyde 3-phosphate. The dihydroxyacetone phosphate produced by the aldolase reaction is, therefore, all converted to glyceraldehyde 3-phosphate before it is further metabolized. Each of the succeeding steps in glycolysis can thus be considered to occur in duplicate. Neither aldolase nor triose phosphate isomerase limits the rate at which glycolysis proceeds.

Glyceraldehyde 3-phosphate is converted to 1,3-diphosphoglyceric acid in a complex reaction catalysed by glyceraldehyde 3-phosphate dehydrogenase and involving the simultaneous conversion of the oxidized form of nicotinamide adenine dinucleotide (NAD^+) to its reduced form NADH and the release of a hydrogen ion. At physiological pH, 1,3-diphosphoglyceric acid exists as the ionized form, 1,3-diphosphoglycerate (1,3-DPG). As well as accepting a hydrogen ion, NAD^+ also accepts two electrons. The additional phosphate group incorporated into 1,3-DPG is derived from inorganic phosphate, so there is no further input of ATP.

The next step in glycolysis is a kinase reaction in which a phosphate group is transferred from 1,3-DPG to ADP. ATP is formed and the 1,3-DPG is converted to 3-phosphoglycerate in a reaction catalysed by phosphoglycerate kinase.

Internal re-organization of the 3-phosphoglycerate molecule shifts the phosphate group to the 2-carbon position, to form 2-phosphoglycerate, in a reaction catalysed by phosphoglyceromutase. A dehydration reaction then occurs, catalysed by enolase, which results in the formation of phosphoenolpyruvate (PEP).

The last step in glycolysis results in the transfer of the phosphate group from phosphoenolpyruvate to ADP, with the formation of ATP and pyruvate. This is another kinase reaction, this time catalysed by pyruvate kinase.

Thus the net effect of glycolysis can be seen to be the conversion of one molecule of glucose to two molecules of pyruvate, with the net formation of two molecules of ATP and the conversion of two molecules of NAD^+ to NADH. If glycogen rather than glucose is the starting point, three molecules of ATP are produced, as there is no initial investment of ATP when the first phosphorylation step occurs. Although this net energy yield appears to be small, the relatively large carbohydrate store available and the rapid rate at which glycolysis can proceed mean that the energy that can be supplied in this way is crucial for the performance of intense exercise. The 800 m runner, for example, obtains about 60% of the total energy requirement from anaerobic metabolism, and may convert about 100 g of carbohydrate (mostly glycogen, and equivalent to about 0.55 moles of glucose) to lactate in less than 2 min. The amount of ATP released in this way (three ATP molecules per glucose molecule degraded, about 1667 mmol of ATP in total) far exceeds that available from phosphocreatine (PCr) hydrolysis. This high rate of anaerobic metabolism allows not only a faster 'steady state' speed than would be possible if aerobic metabolism alone had to be relied upon, but also allows a faster pace in the early stages before the cardiovascular system has adjusted to the demands, and the delivery and utilization of oxygen have increased in response to the exercise stimulus.

The reactions of glycolysis occur in the cytoplasm of the cell, and the pyruvate formed is not phosphorylated and is, therefore, free to leave the cell. Some pyruvate will escape from tissues such as muscle when the rate of glycolysis is high, but most is further metabolized. The fate of the pyruvate produced by glycolysis during exercise will depend not only on factors such as exercise intensity, but also on the metabolic capacity of the tissue.

3.4 Regeneration of NAD^+

When glycolysis proceeds rapidly, the problem for the cell is that the availability of NAD^+, which is necessary as a co-factor in the glyceraldehyde 3-phosphate dehydrogenase reaction, becomes limiting. The amount of NAD^+ in the cell is very small—only about 0.8 mmoles per kg of muscle—relative to the rate at which glycolysis can proceed. In intense activity such as sprinting, the rate of turnover of ATP can be about 125 mmoles per kg of muscle per minute, and in brief bursts of activity induced by electrical stimulation, it can reach 150 mmoles kg^{-1} min^{-1}. If the NADH formed by glycolysis is not reoxidized to NAD^+ at an equal rate, glycolysis will be unable to proceed and to contribute to energy supply.

There are two processes available to most—but not all—cells by which the oxidation of NADH and the regeneration of NAD^+ can occur. Reduction of pyruvate to lactate (Fig. 3.5) will achieve this, and this reaction has the advantage that it can proceed in the absence of oxygen. Lactate can accumulate within the muscle cells, reaching much higher concentrations than those reached by any of the glycolytic intermediates, but when this happens the associated hydrogen ions cause the intracellular pH to fall. Some lactate will diffuse into the extracellular space and will eventually begin to accumulate in the blood. The lactate that leaves the muscle cell is accompanied by hydrogen ions, and this has the effect of making the buffer capacity of the extracellular space available to handle some of the hydrogen ions that would otherwise cause the intracellular pH to fall to a point where it would interfere with cell function. The normal pH of the muscle cell at rest is about 7.1, but this can fall to about 6.5, or even less, in high-intensity exercise when large amounts of lactate are formed. Because some of the hydrogen ions are buffered by the intracellular and extracellular buffers, the increase in lactate and the decrease in pH are not linearly related.

At pH 6.5, the contractile mechanism begins to fail, and some inhibition of key enzymes, such as phosphorylase and phosphofructokinase, may occur. A low pH also stimulates free nerve endings in the muscle, resulting in the perception of pain. Although the negative effects of the acidosis resulting from lactate accumulation are often stressed, it must be remembered that the energy made available by anaerobic glycolysis allows the performance of high-intensity exercise that would otherwise be impossible.

As an alternative to conversion to lactate, pyruvate may undergo oxidative metabolism to carbon dioxide (CO_2) and water. This process occurs within the mitochondrion, and pyruvate is transported across the mitochondrial membrane

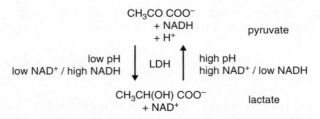

Fig. 3.5 The lactate dehydrogenase reaction catalyses the interconversion of lactate and pyruvate, and can proceed in either direction.

by a specific carrier protein. The first step that occurs within the mitochondrion is the conversion, by oxidative decarboxylation, of the 3-carbon pyruvate to a 2-carbon acetate group which is linked by a thioester bond to coenzyme A to form acetyl-CoA. This reaction, in which NAD^+ is converted to NADH, is catalysed by the pyruvate dehydrogenase enzyme complex.

Acetyl-CoA is oxidized to CO_2 and water in the tricarboxylic acid (TCA) cycle: this series of reactions is also known as the Krebs' cycle, after Hans Krebs who first described the reactions involved, or the citric acid cycle, as citrate is one of the key intermediates in the process. The reactions involve the combination of acetyl-CoA with oxaloacetate to form citrate, a 6-carbon tri-carboxylic acid. A series of reactions leads to the sequential loss of hydrogen ions and carbon dioxide, resulting in the regeneration of oxaloacetate. Acetyl-CoA is also an intermediate of fatty acid oxidation, and the final steps of oxidative degradation are, therefore, common to both fat and carbohydrate. The TCA cycle has been described in more detail in Chapter 1.

In terms of the energy conservation of glucose metabolism, the overall reaction, starting with glucose as the fuel, can be summarized as follows:

$$\text{Glucose} + 6O_2 + 38ADP + 38P_i \rightarrow 6CO_2 + 6H_2O + 38ATP.$$

The total ATP synthesis of 38 moles per mole of glucose oxidized are accounted for primarily by the oxidation of reduced coenzymes in the terminal respiratory system as follows:

ATP synthesized	Source
2	Glycolysis
6	NADH by glycolysis
24	NADH
4	$FADH_2$
2	GTP

One potential problem with the oxidative regeneration of NAD^+ is that the reactions of oxidative phosphorylation occur within the mitochondria, whereas glycolysis is a cytosolic process, and the inner mitochondrial membrane is impermeable to NADH and to NAD^+. Without regeneration of the NAD^+ in the cytoplasm, glycolysis will stop so there must be a mechanism for the effective oxidation of the NADH formed during glycolysis. This separation is overcome by a number of substrate shuttles which transfer reducing equivalents into the mitochondrion.

Some of the pyruvate formed may be converted to the amino acid alanine, and this will be described in Chapter 5. Some may also be converted to the 4-carbon compound oxaloacetate by the incorporation of CO_2 in a reaction catalysed by pyruvate carboxylase, but this reaction does not occur in skeletal muscle due to the absence of pyruvate carboxylase. This conversion to oxaloacetate can be the first step in the resynthesis of glucose by the process of gluconeogenesis. Alternatively, this may be important as an anaplerotic reaction: these are reactions which maintain the intracellular concentration of crucial intermediates which might otherwise become depleted.

3.5 Regulation of glycolysis

The rate of glycolysis must be regulated to ensure that the supply of ATP is matched with the rate of ATP hydrolysis and with the availability of other energy sources. As well as this local regulation within each cell, there is a need for a coherent response in the different tissues involved in carbohydrate metabolism, and for a co-ordination of the pathways of carbohydrate metabolism with those of fat and protein. Regulation is, therefore, complex, and is achieved by the integration of the effects of a number of signals.

There are a number of key steps in carbohydrate metabolism. These include the entry of glucose itself into the cell, which is regulated by a number of factors. The initial phosphorylation by hexokinase (in the case of blood glucose) or phosphorylase (in the case of glycogen) effectively traps the glucose molecule within the muscle cell. The pyruvate dehydrogenase reaction is also crucial since it commits the pyruvate formed by glycolysis to oxidation or to conversion to fat: acetyl-CoA cannot be used for the resynthesis of glucose.

The uptake of glucose from the blood into cells is dependent on the activity of a specific glucose transport protein located in the cell membrane. These receptors are tissue specific, that located in skeletal muscle being GLUT 4. Transport of glucose into cells is generally stimulated by insulin, which promotes storage after carbohydrate-containing meals. Transport into muscle is also stimulated by exercise, increasing the availability of glucose as a substrate.

Regulation of the rate at which glycolysis proceeds can occur at three points in the pathway. The first of these is at the entry point, involving the hexokinase

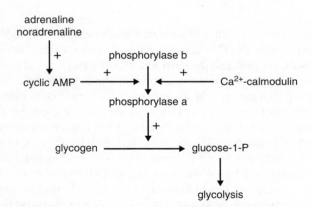

Fig. 3.6 Glycogen breakdown is regulated by the action of the catecholamines and by local stimulation by calcium.

or phosphorylase reaction. Hexokinase activity is stimulated by inorganic phosphate, one of the reaction substrates, and is inhibited by the reaction product glucose 6-phosphate. The regulation of phosphorylase is more complex (Fig. 3.6). The enzyme exists in two forms: these are designated phosphorylase a and phosphorylase b. Phosphorylase a has a much higher activity, and is referred to as the active form of the enzyme, although the b form does have some activity. Phosphorylase b is converted to the a form by the enzyme phosphorylase kinase, which adds a phosphate group derived from ATP. Conversion to the b form is promoted by a phosphatase enzyme which removes the phosphate group from phosphorylase a. Phosphorylase kinase itself also exists in active (a) and inactive (b) forms, the activation being promoted by a protein kinase. The activity of this protein kinase, in turn, is stimulated by the action of adrenaline: the action of adrenaline at the cell surface increases the intracellular cyclic AMP concentration, and this, in turn, stimulates the protein kinase activity. At times of stress, the circulating adrenaline concentration increases, leading to a large increase in phosphorylase a activity. This will only result in a high rate of glycogenolysis if the intracellular calcium concentration is high: this mechanism prevents the rapid breakdown of glycogen at rest, when energy is not needed, but allows high rates of glycogenolysis during exercise when activation of the muscles increases the free calcium concentration within the cell. As calcium initiates the contractile process, as well as binding to calmodulin and thus activating protein kinase, this ensures a close coupling between muscle activity and substrate supply. High levels of insulin have no effect on the intracellular cyclic AMP concentration in skeletal muscle, but will inactivate phosphorylase and reduce the rate of glycogenolysis. As high insulin levels generally occur only after carbohydrate feeding, this tends to favour storage of ingested carbohydrate. During exercise, phosphorylase a activity is high at the onset of exercise, but there is then a reversion to the b form: in spite of this, and for reasons not well understood, a high rate of glycogenolysis continues. Activation of the b form, which does have some catalytic activity in the presence of inosine monophosphate (IMP), formed by the breakdown of ATP, may be one important factor.

Phosphofructokinase (PFK) is a key regulatory enzyme, the activity of which is modified by many different compounds, although not all of these appear to be of physiological significance. Of crucial importance is the fact that PFK activity is inhibited by high ATP and PCr levels in the cell and stimulated by high levels of ADP and AMP: this means that the activity is low when the cell is energy-replete, but is high when the energy charge of the cell is low (Fig. 3.7). Citrate has been shown to be an inhibitor of PFK, at least in isolated preparations, and citrate accumulation within the muscle cell may also inhibit the activity of PFK; this mechanism provides a potential link for the integration of fat and carbohydrate metabolism. A high rate of fatty acid oxidation results in citrate accumulation within the mitochondrion: some of this will be transported into the cytoplasm, resulting in a reduction in the rate of glycolysis. Inhibition of PFK will also cause the accumulation of G6-P, which will inhibit the activity of

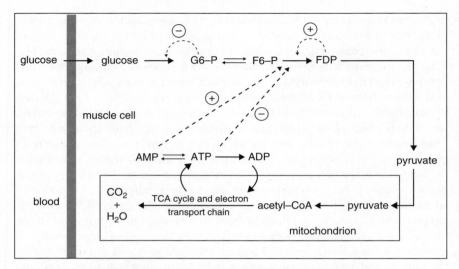

Fig. 3.7 Phosphofructokinase plays a key role in regulating the rate of glycolysis, and is responsive to changes in the energy charge of the cell. If the concentration of AMP rises, PFK activity is increased: a high ATP concentration has an inhibitory effect, slowing the rate of glycolysis and conserving carbohydrate.

hexokinase, and reduce the entry into the cell of glucose that is not needed. Both the reaction substrate (F6P) and the product (FDP) can activate the enzyme. Other activators include ammonia and inorganic phosphate: the concentration of both these substances will increase at the onset of exercise, and this stimulation of activity may be sufficient to overcome the inhibitory effects of the fall in pH which is normally observed at this time. Some of these key steps in the regulation of carbohydrate degradation are shown in Fig. 3.8. The integrated metabolic response to exercise is discussed in more detail in Chapters 6 and 7.

Pyruvate kinase activity is regulated by some of the same factors that affect PFK activity: these include activation by high ADP concentrations and inhibition by both ATP and PCr.

Pyruvate dehydrogenase (PDH) is not a single enzyme, but is a complex of three enzymes which can exist in an active (a) dephosphorylated form and an inactive (b) phosphorylated form. Control of the activity of this enzyme complex is central to the integration of the metabolic response to exercise, but the control mechanisms are not well understood. As with other similar enzymes, interconversion is modulated by specific kinase and phosphatase reactions. Regulation of the activity of the enzyme complex can, therefore, be achieved by modification of the activity of the interconverting enzymes, which will determine the amount of the active form of the enzyme. In skeletal muscle, exercise will result in an increase in the concentration of pyruvate and of calcium, a

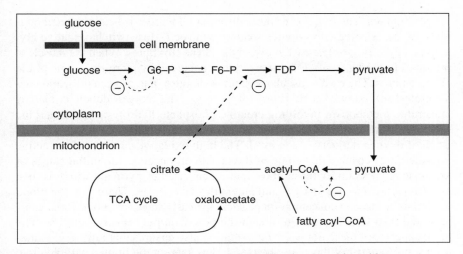

Fig. 3.8 Integration of fat and carbohydrate utilization is achieved by co-ordination at a number of steps.

decrease in the ATP/ADP ratio, an increase in the NADH/NAD$^+$ ratio, and a decrease in the acetyl-CoA/CoA-SH ratio (CoA-SH is the free form of CoA). All these factors will tend to increase the amount of the PDH complex present in the active form due to the effects of the interconverting enzymes.

Hormonal influences extend the regulation of CHO metabolism beyond the boundaries of the cell and allow integration of the responses of the different tissues involved. This is discussed in detail below.

3.6 Carbohydrate utilization in different tissues

Some tissues, most notably the red blood cells, but also the renal medulla and the retina, have no mitochondria and, therefore, no capacity for oxidative metabolism. Hence, these tissues are obliged to rely solely on glycolysis for energy production. Most tissues, however, can use a variety of fuels and have the option of anaerobic or aerobic metabolism.

Skeletal muscle is a good example of a tissue that can derive most of its energy requirement from oxidative metabolism or from anaerobic metabolism, and the choice of fuel depends on a number of factors, including the metabolic capacity of the tissue, the availability of substrate, and the availability of oxygen. Although the conversion of glucose to lactate is an anaerobic process, it occurs even when oxygen is freely available to the muscle, and lactate release does not necessarily imply that the oxygen supply is inadequate.

Skeletal muscle contains two main fibre types (Type I and Type II) as described in Chapter 1. The Type II fibres can be subdivided into Type IIa and

Type IIb fibres. The function of these different fibre types is better understood if they are described as slow-twitch oxidative (Type I), fast-twitch oxidative glycolytic (Type IIa), or fast-twitch glycolytic (Type IIb) fibres. When the muscle is required to produce only low forces, this is achieved by recruiting some of the Type 1 fibres. The cardiovascular system is sluggish, and oxygen utilization accelerates only slowly at the onset of exercise: the oxygen deficit is met by anaerobic metabolism involving creatine phosphate hydrolysis and anaerobic glycolysis. After the initial one or two minutes of exercise, however, a steady state of oxygen delivery is achieved. The high oxidative capacity of the active muscle fibres ensures that some of the lactate produced in the initial stages of exercise is taken up by these fibres and reconverted to pyruvate which is then decarboxylated to acetyl-CoA and enters the TCA cycle. Therefore, the blood (and muscle) lactate concentration peaks in the early stages of submaximal exercise and then falls later, even though the power output remains constant. The high capacity of these fibres for fat oxidation also ensures that fatty acid oxidation supplies most of the energy demand, thus sparing the limited carbohydrate reserves. When carbohydrate is used by these fibres, it will normally be oxidized completely to carbon dioxide and water, thus maximizing the ATP return.

At higher force requirements, the muscle begins to recruit some of the Type II fibres: first the Type IIa fibres, and then at higher forces the Type IIb fibres. The oxygen consumption increases as work output increases, indicating an increasing rate of oxidative metabolism, but as the active fibres begin to include those with a high activity of glycolytic enzymes relative to the activity of the oxidative enzymes, a point is reached where, in these fibres, the rate of pyruvate formation by glycolysis exceeds the rate at which the pyruvate can enter the TCA cycle. The excess pyruvate must, therefore, be reduced to lactate to allow regeneration of the NAD^+ and continued flux through the glycolytic pathway. At these high work rates, the blood lactate concentration rises progressively throughout exercise, and the work time is necessarily short as fatigue supervenes. Lactate production will thus occur, even when there is no restriction on the oxygen availability to the muscle cells: the accumulation of lactate in the blood is, therefore, largely a reflection of the activation of muscle fibres in which the glycolytic capacity exceeds the capacity for the oxidative metabolism of pyruvate. The differing capacities of the different fibre types in human skeletal muscle for carbohydrate breakdown is indicated by the differences in phosphorylase activity in these fibres: the activity is higher in Type IIb fibres (8.8 U g^{-1}) than in Type IIa (5.8 U g^{-1}) or Type I (2.8 U g^{-1}) fibres (Essen *et al.* 1976).

The differing enzyme activities of the different skeletal muscle fibre types offer the opportunity for an exchange of carbohydrate substrate between muscles or between fibres within the same muscle: if the Type II fibres are recruited and release lactate into the extracellular space, this might be taken up and oxidized by the adjacent Type I fibres, which have a high oxidative capacity. Because of this uptake, some of the lactate formed by glycolysis during exercise will not appear in the blood. Cardiac muscle can be regarded as a type of muscle with an extremely high oxidative capacity and a low glycolytic capacity, and will use lactate as a fuel for oxidation if this is available from the blood.

The liver plays a central role in carbohydrate homeostasis. It acts as a glycogen reservoir: the presence of the enzyme glucose 6-phosphatase allows free glucose to be released from the cell for the maintenance of the blood glucose concentration. The high capacity of liver tissue for gluconeogenesis also allows the liver to play a major role in providing glucose for the brain and other obligatory glucose users in times of starvation or CHO deprivation. Even during short periods of starvation, as in the normal overnight fast, the liver glycogen content falls markedly and gluconeogenesis is accelerated. After exercise, if the blood lactate has been elevated, the liver will remove a large part of this and will use it to resynthesize glucose.

3.7 Gluconeogenesis: formation of glucose from non-carbohydrate sources

After exercise, the liver and muscle glycogen stores will be depleted, the extent of the depletion depending on a number of factors including mainly the duration and intensity of the exercise. In very high-intensity exercise where fatigue occurs within a few minutes, a large part of the glycogen store in the exercising muscles will have been converted to lactate, although the glycogen content of the resting muscles will remain intact. There will also be little depletion of liver glycogen. If the exercise is prolonged (1–2 h), and is continued to the point of fatigue, both the liver and the muscle glycogen, stores may be almost completely depleted. Chapters 6 and 7 describe these effects in detail.

Replenishment of the muscle and liver glycogen stores is an essential part of the recovery process. In the absence of dietary carbohydrate intake, some resynthesis can take place using non-carbohydrate sources, but an intake of carbohydrate-containing foods is essential for complete recovery. Nutritional factors influencing the recovery of liver and muscle glycogen stores will be considered in Chapter 7. Gluconeogenesis—the synthesis of glucose from non-glucose sources—allows some recovery even in the absence of food intake, but also becomes important during starvation by making glucose available to those tissues which cannot use any other fuel. Gluconeogenesis also allows recycling of the lactate produced by tissues such as red blood cells: the body's total lactate turnover per day may exceed 100 g, and lactate losses from the body in sweat and urine are extremely small.

A variety of substrates can contribute to the process of gluconeogenesis (Fig. 3.9). Lactate and pyruvate produced by glycolysis can be used, as well as the glycerol backbone of triglyceride molecules and the carbon skeletons of some amino acids. After high-intensity exercise, the circulating lactate concentration will be high. If gentle exercise is performed at this time some of this lactate will be used as a fuel for oxidation by the Type I muscle fibres which are primarily active in low-intensity exercise, and some lactate will also be taken up from the circulation and oxidized by the heart. If the individual rests after exercise, the rate of energy expenditure is low, and there is no need for energy production by oxidation of the circulating lactate, and in this situation most of it will be re-converted to glucose.

Gluconeogenesis takes place mostly in the liver, and to a lesser extent in the kidney. There has been some debate as to how far this process can proceed in mammalian skeletal muscle, but it seems that this can take place to some extent, using lactate as a starting point, if the muscle glycogen content is low and the lactate concentration is high, as may occur after exercise. The reactions of gluconeogenesis involve the reversal of the reactions of glycolysis, where this is possible, but the irreversible reactions must be by-passed by a different route. Gluconeogenesis is an energy-demanding process, and can take place only when ATP is available to the cell.

The irreversible reactions of glycolysis and the means by which they are by-passed are:

Enzyme	Reaction	By-pass enzyme
Hexokinase	Glucose → G6P	Glucose 6-phosphatase
Phosphofructokinase	F6P → FDP	FDPase
Pyruvate kinase	PEP → Pyruvate	Pyruvate carboxylase + Phosphoenolpyruvate phosphokinase

Glycerol can contribute to gluconeogenesis in prolonged exercise when the rate of fat oxidation, and therefore of triglyceride hydrolysis, is relatively high. In quantitative terms, however, the contribution of glycerol to glucose homeostasis during exercise is small. In other situations, such as in prolonged fasting, glycerol plays a major role in maintaining the availability of glucose for those tissues where it is essential: about 20 g of glycerol per day is released as the body's fat stores are mobilized, and most of this is converted to glucose. Gluconeogenesis of glycerol proceeds by uptake into the hepatocytes (the liver cells): glycerol is a small molecule and appears to diffuse readily.

Glycerol kinase phosphorylates the glycerol inside the cell to form glycerol 3-phosphate, using one molecule of ATP in the process, and the glycerol 3-phosphate so formed is converted to dihydroxyacetone phosphate in an $NAD^+/NADH$-dependent reaction catalysed by glycerol 3-phosphate dehydrogenase. The dihydroxyacetone phosphate can then enter the glycolytic pathway and be used for gluconeogenesis. It is clear that these reactions can only occur when sufficient ATP is available to the cell and when the reduced/oxidized ratio of NAD^+ permits.

The carbon skeletons of most amino acids can contribute to glucose synthesis, and these amino acids are referred to as glucogenic. These amino acids can be metabolized to pyruvate or to intermediates of the TCA cycle, and can then be used for glucose synthesis. Metabolism of two amino acids (leucine and lysine)

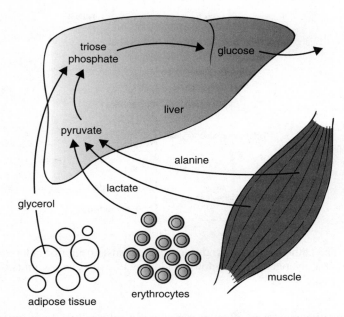

Fig. 3.9 Gluconeogenesis takes place primarily in the liver, using lactate, glycerol, and amino acids released from other tissues.

results in the formation of acetyl-CoA, but there is no mechanism by which this can be converted to glucose, although ketone body synthesis is possible: these amino acids are referred to as ketogenic. Protein oxidation during exercise can make only a small contribution to energy production, but gluconeogenesis allows the large energy store tied up in non-essential body protein to contribute to the maintenance of blood glucose during prolonged fasting. Amino acid metabolism is described further in Chapter 5.

3.8 Glycogen synthesis

Replenishment of the carbohydrate stores of liver and muscle requires that glucose derived from the diet, as well as that resulting from gluconeogenesis, be used for glycogen resynthesis. The common intermediate, whether glycogenesis is occurring from glucose taken up from the blood or is the result of gluconeogenesis, is glucose 6-phosphate. The former is much more likely in muscle, but either source is possible in liver. The G6P is then converted to glucose 1-phosphate by the action of phosphoglucomutase. Uridine triphosphate (UTP) then reacts with the G1P to form UDP-glucose and pyrophosphate (PPi) in a reaction catalysed by glucose 1-phosphate uridyltransferase (Fig. 3.10). The glucose residue is then attached by an α-1,4 glycosidic bond to the free end of a

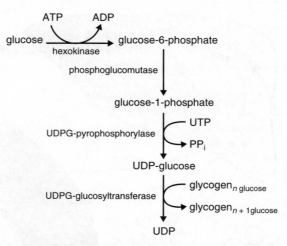

Fig. 3.10 The pathway for the synthesis of glycogen starting from glucose. It is assumed that a glycogen skeleton for the addition of extra glucose units is always available.

pre-existing glycogen molecule: this reaction is catalysed by glycogen synthase. The branch points are introduced into the glycogen structure by the activity of a branching enzyme: when the length of an end chain is about 12 glucose residues long, this enzyme detaches a chain about 7 residues long and re-attaches it to a neighbouring chain by an α-1,6 bond.

The activity of glycogen synthase is crucial to the process of glycogen synthesis, and this enzyme, like many others, exists in active (glycogen synthase a: non-phosphorylated) and relatively inactive (glycogen synthase b: phosphorylated) forms, with the interconversions catalysed by specific enzymes.

Hormonal control of glycogen synthase is exerted by adrenaline, which activates the protein kinase and converts the synthase into the inactive form, and by insulin which promotes glycogen synthesis. At a local level, increasing calcium levels, seen during contraction, reduce glycogen synthase activity.

Restoration of the liver and muscle glycogen stores is an important part of the recovery process after prolonged exercise. Where adequate dietary carbohydrate is available, replenishment of the stores normally requires about 24–36 h, with the synthesis rate in the initial period being faster in Type I than in Type II muscle fibres. Glycogen synthetic rates are critically dependent on the carbohydrate content of the diet, and restriction of the carbohydrate intake will prevent restoration of normal, tissue glycogen stores. The highest rates of glycogen synthesis are achieved if a high-carbohydrate meal is consumed immediately after the end of prolonged exercise. Delaying carbohydrate ingestion for even 2 h can prevent the maximal rates of resynthesis from occurring. The high rates of glucose uptake into the muscle, observed during exercise, continue for some time after exercise and provide the substrate for glycogen resynthesis.

Feeding of fructose after exercise favours resynthesis of the liver glycogen store, and will not allow optimum replacement of the muscle glycogen, whereas glucose feeding seems to favour replacement of the muscle glycogen stores. Sucrose should allow replacement of both of these carbohydrate reserves.

3.9 Hormonal control of carbohydrate metabolism

A number of hormones play crucial roles in regulating the rate of carbohydrate utilization, as well as in integrating the supply and utilization of carbohydrate fuels in different tissues at rest and during exercise. The blood glucose concentration must be maintained within narrow limits, and cannot be allowed to rise too far after a high-carbohydrate meal or to fall too far, even though the rate of uptake by the exercising muscles may increase many fold. Equally, the muscle glycogen stores are essential fuels during exercise, but they are present in only a limited amount and must be conserved. The integrated metabolic response to exercise will be discussed in detail in Chapters 6 and 7, but the hormonal factors which influence carbohydrate metabolism will be described briefly here. Because the effects on carbohydrate cannot be considered in isolation, the effects on other metabolic processes will also be briefly covered below.

Insulin, a polypeptide hormone consisting of two peptide chains (an A Chain of 21 amino acids and a B chain of 30 amino acids) plays a key role in the regulation of carbohydrate metabolism, and because it also has a regulatory function in lipid and protein metabolism its role can be seen as central to the body's fuel homeostasis. Secretion of insulin by the β cells of the Islets of Langerhans in the pancreas is stimulated by an increasing blood glucose concentration (Fig. 3.11). In both skeletal and cardiac muscle, the effect of increasing insulin concentrations is to increase the number of active glucose transporters and thus stimulate the membrane transport of glucose. Glycogen synthase is also activated by the action of insulin on the protein phosphatase enzyme which regulates the interconversion of the active and inactive forms of glycogen synthase. In contrast to the situation in muscle, insulin has no effect on glucose transport

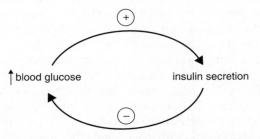

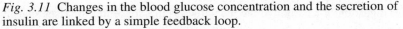

Fig. 3.11 Changes in the blood glucose concentration and the secretion of insulin are linked by a simple feedback loop.

in the liver since the hepatic cell membranes are freely permeable to glucose. However, it does increase the activity of glucokinase, which phosphorylates glucose entering the cells, and there is also some evidence that it increases glycogen synthesis, by activating glycogen synthase, thus tending to promote glucose storage. It also reduces the rate of hepatic gluconeogenesis, and decreases glycogenolysis by inhibiting phosphorylase. Glucose uptake into the brain and its subsequent metabolism in nervous tissue is insensitive to insulin.

The catecholamines, adrenaline and noradrenaline, have many cardiovascular and metabolic effects. The secretions of the adrenal medulla consist of about 80% adrenaline and 20% noradrenaline, but noradrenaline released from sympathetic nerve endings can also appear in the circulation. In response to exercise and other stresses, the circulating catecholamine concentrations increase. At the cell membrane, adrenaline activates the membrane-bound enzyme adenyl cyclase, resulting in an increase in the rate of cyclic AMP formation within the target cell. An increase in the intracellular cyclic AMP concentration causes an activation of phosphorylase and an increased rate of glycogen breakdown in active muscle: stimulation of glycogenolysis in resting muscle is largely prevented because of the low, intracellular free-calcium levels. The catecholamines also stimulate glycogenolysis in the liver and lipolysis in adipose tissue, effectively mobilizing fuels that the muscles can use.

The actions of glucagon, a single-chain polypeptide containing 29 amino acids which is also secreted by the pancreas, are generally antagonistic to those of insulin: it is the concentration ratio of these two hormones that determines their integrated effect on fuel mobilization. The effects of increased glucagon concentration are to stimulate glycogenolysis and gluconeogenesis in the liver, increasing the availability of blood glucose, and to stimulate lipolysis in adipose tissue, thereby increasing the availability of free fatty acids (FFA) for uptake by the muscle.

Several other hormones and peptides also play important roles in fuel mobilization. Growth hormone, released from the anterior pituitary gland, promotes protein synthesis, but also stimulates gluconeogenesis in the liver and decreases peripheral glucose uptake. Growth hormone also stimulates lipolysis in adipose tissue, but this effect is observed only in the presence of glucocorticoids. Cortisol is a glucocorticoid hormone released from the adrenal cortex, and many of its diverse actions involve a potentiation of the effect of other hormones: it increases the gluconeogenic response of the liver in the presence of adrenaline and glucagon and also increases the lipolytic rate in adipose tissue in the presence of adrenaline and growth hormone. The thyroid hormones triiodothyronine and thyroxine generally act to stimulate the mobilization of fuels.

Because of the number of possible regulatory factors involved and the interactions of these factors, the hormonal and metabolic response to any metabolic disturbance, such as food ingestion or exercise, is complex, involving a number of different tissues as well as different control processes.

After ingestion of a carbohydrate meal, the insulin concentration rises sharply to promote the disposal of the glucose which appears in the blood, and the

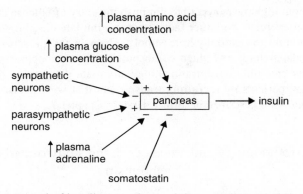

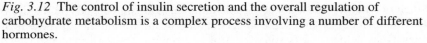

Fig. 3.12 The control of insulin secretion and the overall regulation of carbohydrate metabolism is a complex process involving a number of different hormones.

glucagon concentration falls. Insulin release occurs in response to the changing blood glucose concentration which is monitored by the β cells of the pancreas, and thus forms part of a simple feedback loop (Fig. 3.11). The action of this feedback system is more complex, however, as changing plasma amino acid levels also influence insulin output; the pancreas is also affected by plasma adrenaline levels, which have a powerful inhibitory effect on insulin release, as well as by the circulating concentration of other hormones and by the activity of its sympathetic and parasympathetic nerve supply (Fig. 3.12). In response to food intake, a large number of small peptides are released by the intestine and some of these act to stimulate insulin secretion. Increases in the circulating levels of glucose, amino acids, and fatty acids (for example, after a mixed meal) stimulate the output of somatostatin, a small (14 amino acids) peptide from the δ cells of the pancreas. Somatostatin acts locally within the pancreas to inhibit insulin release, thus providing a brake which prevents excessive insulin secretion. In addition, it also reduces gastrointestinal motility and secretion of digestive juices, hence slowing the absorption of food. The glycogen synthetic pathway is activated in muscle and in liver. Fatty acid mobilization from adipose tissue is suppressed and the rate of amino acid breakdown is also decreased. Anabolic reactions are, therefore, promoted and catabolic reactions suppressed.

In the early stages of prolonged exercise, the uptake of FFA from the plasma is increased, probably because of the increased plasma flow through the muscle capillary bed, and therefore, the circulating FFA concentration falls. As exercise proceeds, the plasma levels of adrenaline, noradrenaline, glucagon, cortisol, and growth hormone all increase, whereas the secretion of insulin is suppressed: increases in the circulating catecholamine concentration have a powerful inhibitory effect on insulin release as well as activating phosphorylase and stimulating lipolysis. These changes promote FFA release from adipose tissue, increasing the plasma FFA concentration and hence increasing their uptake and oxidation by the exercising muscles. The fall in the circulating insulin concentration might be expected to diminish the entry of glucose into the muscle cells during exercise, but other factors act to stimulate the glucose transporters and to maintain the carbohydrate supply. Even in the presence of very low insulin levels, high rates of glucose transport occur, and it appears that increased intracellular calcium concentrations may stimulate the activity of the glucose transporters, perhaps by recruiting transporters that were previously inactive. These changes are described in further detail in Chapter 7.

3.10 Methodology and advances in the study of carbohydrate metabolism

Much of what we know about carbohydrate metabolism depends on the use of specific techniques, and some understanding of the limitations of these techniques may help to clarify some areas of uncertainty. The earliest steps taken to elucidate the intermediate steps in the degradation and synthesis of carbohydrates used a variety of isolated cell or subcellular preparations. Loss of structural integrity obviously means some loss of information, for example in the understanding of processes that involve membrane transport. The use of purified enzyme preparations for the study of reaction kinetics may also give results that do not apply in the conditions that prevail in the living cell, so some caution is necessary in the interpretation of these results.

The re-introduction of the needle-biopsy technique for the study of muscle metabolism, which had been developed in the late nineteenth century but had fallen into disuse, allowed enormous steps forward to be made in the 1960s and 1970s. The technique is simple, fairly painless, and without significant risk, and it allows repeated sampling of the major muscle groups. A progressive utilization of the muscle glycogen stores was shown to occur during exercise; studies where only one leg was used in exercise showed that there was little or no change in the glycogen content of the resting muscles. The rate of glycogen utilization was proportional to exercise intensity, increasing exponentially as the power output increased. Depletion of glycogen appeared not to be the cause of fatigue in high-intensity exercise as large amounts of glycogen remained at the point of fatigue. Accumulation of lactate and depletion of creatine phosphate, with only small decreases in the muscle ATP content, were also demonstrated at this time. Recovery of the muscle glycogen store was shown to be rather slow, and also to depend critically on the carbohydrate content of the diet. Histochemical techniques were applied to estimate the changes in glycogen content occurring in the different fibre types. Later, this procedure was refined by the use of dissected individual muscle fibres. These were separated from the freeze-dried biopsy sample, assessed for fibre type, and then subjected to biochemical analysis. These techniques allowed the utilization of glycogen in the different fibre types to be quantified in different exercise situations. However, there are some limitations to the use of the biopsy technique: where serial samples are taken for the study of carbohydrate metabolism, successive samples should be taken in the proximal direction, and should be separated by at least 2.5 cm from the preceding sample sites since the sampling procedure itself will disturb the normal pattern of metabolism.

The biopsy technique has been used with limited success to quantify the utilization of local fat stores during exercise. Some fat is stored within the muscle fibre as lipid droplets, and some as adipose cells between muscle fibres. The biopsy technique, however, does not readily distinguish between these two different fat depots.

In a limited number of studies, a modification of the muscle-biopsy technique has been used to take samples from the livers of healthy volunteers, and changes in the storage of glycogen with exercise and diet have been demonstrated. The technique is not without some risk of bleeding, and unlike the muscle, it is not easy to apply pressure to stop bleeding.

Tracer methods involving a variety of different isotopic labels have been used to assess the contributions of different fuels to substrate utilization in a variety of exercise models. Constant-rate infusions of labelled glucose in trace amounts have been used to assess the appearance of glucose derived from the liver in the bloodstream, and the appearance of labelled carbon atoms in the expired carbon dioxide gives an indication of the oxidation rate of the blood glucose. The oxidation of ingested carbohydrates can be followed in the same way. Separation of labelled intermediates from blood and muscle allows the metabolic fate of administered tracers to be established. These methods have provided valuable insights into the rates of oxidation of different substrates in exercise.

Tissue or organ metabolism has been studied by measuring concentration differences in arterial and venous blood across the tissue: if tissue blood flow is also known, quantitative measures of substrate exchange can be obtained. By cannulating the femoral artery and the femoral vein, which drains the quadriceps muscles at the front of the thigh, the oxygen and substrate extraction and metabolite release from these muscles can be studied at rest and during exercise. The technique can be applied in conjunction with isotopic labelling to provide further information.

New developments in magnetic resonance spectroscopy have provided opportunities for the biochemist to study metabolism in the intact organism in a way that was previously impossible. This technique allows the non-invasive estimation of changes in the tissue concentrations of glycogen, PCr, ATP, ADP, AMP, and of changes in tissue pH.

In practice, the picture that we have of the biochemical response to exercise is based on information from all available sources. With further refinement of these methods, new insights will be obtained.

Key points

1. Carbohydrate is normally the largest part of the dietary energy intake (about 40–60% of total energy intake), but the body carbohydrate stores are small: about 80–110 g of glycogen is stored in the liver and about 250–400 g in the muscles.

2. Carbohydrate is used to provide energy by anaerobic metabolism, with lactate as the end-product, or by complete oxidation to carbon dioxide and water. The net effect of glycolysis is to convert one molecule of glucose to two molecules of pyruvate: this process makes two molecules of ATP available for each molecule of glucose broken down. If muscle glycogen is the starting substrate, three ATP molecules are generated for each glucose residue passing down the pathway.

3. Glycolysis involves the reduction of NAD^+ to NADH, resulting in depletion of the intracellular pool of NAD^+. Reduction of pyruvate to lactate allows the NAD^+ to be regenerated from NADH. The alternative pathway for NAD^+ regeneration involves conversion of pyruvate to acetyl-CoA for subsequent oxidation in the TCA cycle.

4. Lactate will accumulate in the muscle when the rate of anaerobic glycolysis exceeds the rate of flux through the pyruvate dehydrogenase reaction (which converts pyruvate to acetyl-CoA). Lactate accumulation is accompanied by accumulation of hydrogen ions, which may interfere with muscle activation and contraction.

5. The body's limited carbohydrate stores are rapidly depleted during exercise (muscle glycogen) or during fasting (liver glycogen). Muscle glycogen stores are normally depleted after 1–2 h of hard exercise. In very high-intensity exercise, the muscle glycogen content falls rapidly, but is not completely depleted at the point of fatigue.

6. Carbohydrate is the major fuel for muscle activity in high-intensity exercise: when the muscle glycogen stores are depleted, only low-intensity exercise is possible. The time for which a fixed exercise intensity can be sustained is related to the size of the pre-exercise glycogen store. This will depend on the pattern of exercise and diet in the previous hours and days.

7. Gluconeogenesis—the synthesis of carbohydrate from non-carbohydrate sources—occurs primarily in the liver, and can help maintain the carbohydrate supply to tissues such as the brain and red blood cells which are dependent on the availability of glucose.

8. A number of hormones are involved in the integration and control of carbohydrate metabolism, including especially insulin, which promotes carbohydrate storage, and glucagon, whose actions are generally antagonistic to those of insulin. Adrenaline and noradrenaline stimulate carbohydrate mobilization and metabolism at times of stress.

Further reading

Boobis, L. H. (1987). Metabolic aspects of sprinting. In: *Exercise: benefits, limits and adaptations* (ed. D. A. D. Macleod *et al*, pp. 116–40. Spon, London.

Costill, D. L. and Miller, J. M. (1980). Nutrition for endurance sport: Carbohydrate and fluid balance. *Int. J. Sports Med.*, **1**, 2–14.

Maughan, R. J. and Greenhaff, P. L. (1991). High intensity exercise and acid–base balance: the influence of diet and induced metabolic alkalosis on performance. In: *Advances in nutrition and top sport*, (ed. F. Brouns) pp. 147–65. Karger, Basel.

Newsholme, E. A. and Leech, A. R. (1983). *Biochemistry for the medical sciences*. Wiley, Chichester.

Sahlin, K. (1986). Metabolic changes limiting muscle performance. In: *Biochemistry of exercise vi* (ed. B. Saltin), pp. 323–45. Human Kinetics, Champaign, IL.

Sjodin, B. (1992). Anaerobic function. *Sport Sci. Rev.* **1**, 13–27.

References

Essen, B., Jansson, E., Henriksson, J., Taylor, A. W., and Saltin, B. (1976). Metabolic characteristics of fibre types in human skeletal muscle. *Acta Physiol. Scand.*, **95**, 153–65.

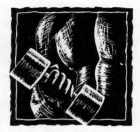

4
Lipid metabolism

4.1 Role of lipids

Lipids or fats contain the same structural elements as carbohydrates, namely carbon, hydrogen, and oxygen, except that the ratio of hydrogen to oxygen is considerably higher in compounds classed as lipids. For example, the common lipid tripalmitin (tripalmitoylglycerol) has the chemical formula $C_{51}H_{98}O_6$. Most lipids can be classified into one of three main types: simple lipids, compound lipids, and derived lipids. Lipids are found in both plant and animal foodstuffs and exhibit generally poor solubility in water. Lipids provide the largest nutrient store of chemical energy that can be used to power biological work, including muscular contraction. Storage depots of lipid in adipose tissue provide insulation from the cold and protect vital organs. Lipids are important structural components of membranes. Dietary lipid also acts as a carrier of the fat-soluble vitamins: A, D, E, and K.

4.2 Types of lipids

Lipids can be classified according to their structure. The three main classes are simple lipids, compound lipids, and derived lipids.

4.2.1 Simple lipids

The simple lipids are often referred to as 'neutral lipids' and consist mainly of triacylglycerols (triglycerides). These are the principal storage form of fat in the body. More than 95% of body fat is triacylglycerol. The majority of this is stored in the cytoplasm of white adipose-tissue cells, although the liver and skeletal muscle also contain stores of important physiological significance. The triacylglycerol molecule (Fig. 4.1) consists of a glycerol 3-carbon molecule backbone attached to which are three molecules of fatty acid. All fatty acids possess a linear hydrocarbon chain and a terminal carboxylic acid group (-COOH). Nearly all have an even number of carbon atoms and are between 14 and 22 carbon atoms long (Table 4.1); those having 16 or 18 atoms are by far the most abundant. Fatty acids may be either saturated or unsaturated. A saturated fatty acid (e.g. palmitic acid) contains carbon atoms joined together by

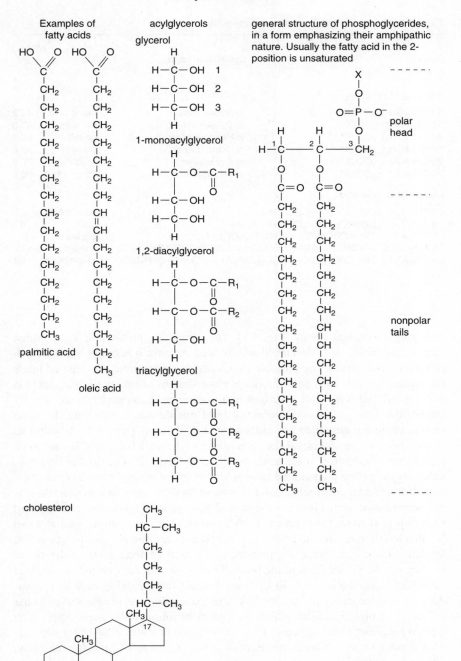

Fig. 4.1 Lipid structures.

Table 4.1   Some naturally occurring fatty acids

Carbon atoms	Structure	Systematic name	Common name	Melting point (°C)
Saturated fatty acids				
12	$CH_3(CH_2)_{10}COOH$	n-Dodecanoic	lauric acid	44.2
14	$CH_3(CH_2)_{12}COOH$	n-Tetradecanoic	myristic	53.9
16	$CH_3(CH_2)_{14}COOH$	n-Hexadecanoic	palmitic	63.1
18	$CH_3(CH_2)_{16}COOH$	n-Octadecanoic	stearic	69.6
20	$CH_3(CH_2)_{18}COOH$	n-Eicosanoic	arachidic	76.5
24	$CH_3(CH_2)_{22}COOH$	n-Tetracosanoic	lignoceric	86.0
Unsaturated fatty acids				
16	$CH_3(CH_2)_5CH{=}CH(CH_2)_7COOH$		palmitoleic	− 0.5
18	$CH_3(CH_2)_7CH{=}CH(CH_2)_7COOH$		oleic	13.4
18	$CH_3(CH_2)_4CH{=}CHCH_2CH{=}CH(CH_2)_7COOH$		linoleic	− 5
18	$CH_3CH_2CH{=}CHCH_2CH{=}CHCH_2CH{=}CH(CH_2)_7COOH$		linolenic	−11
20	$CH_3(CH_2)_4CH{=}CHCH_2CH{=}CHCH_2CH{=}CHCH_2CH{=}CH(CH_2)_3COOH$		arachidonic	−49.5

only single covalent bonds (Fig. 4.1). The remaining bonds link to hydrogen atoms. The molecule is described as saturated because it holds as many hydrogen atoms as is chemically possible. Abundant dietary sources of saturated lipids are meats, egg yolk, and dairy produce. Plant sources of saturated lipids include coconut oil, palm oil, and hydrogenated margarine. Saturated fats are usually semi-solid. Fatty acids that contain at least one double bond along the main carbon chain are classified as unsaturated (Fig. 4.1 and Table 4.1). If only one double bond is present along the carbon chain, then the fatty acid is said to be mono-unsaturated (e.g. oleic acid) as found in olive oil. The double bonds of naturally occurring unsaturated fatty acids are in the *cis* geometrical configuration. If more than one double bond is present then the fatty acid is described as polyunsaturated, as in corn, soyabean, and sunflower oils. Unsaturated fats tend to be liquid at room temperature. Lipids can be obtained from the diet and can be also synthesized in the body. The exceptions are the essential fatty acids, linoleic, linolenic, and arachidonic acid, which must be obtained from the diet as they cannot be synthesized in the body. These essential fatty acids are required for maintaining the integrity of cell membranes, for normal growth and reproduction, and for maintaining a healthy skin. Arachidonic acid also serves as the precursor of prostaglandins which are important intercellular messengers. The typical intake of triacylglycerol in a western diet is about 100–150 g per day. This dietary triacylglycerol represents the major source of lipid for the body, although additional amounts can be synthesized from carbohydrate, particularly when the proportion of carbohydrate in the diet is high and that of triacylglycerol is low.

4.2.2 Compound lipids

These are composed of a neutral fat in combination with other chemicals. The main groups are glycolipids, sphingolipids, phosphoglycerides, and lipoproteins. Glycolipids are diacylglycerols (diglycerides) in which the third hydroxyl group of the glycerol backbone forms a glycoside linkage with a sugar. Sphingolipids contain one molecule of a fatty acid in amide linkage with one molecule of the long-chain unsaturated amino alcohol sphingosine or its saturated analogue dihydrosphingosine, and a polar head group attached at the 1-hydroxyl position of the sphingosine. Sphingolipids do not contain glycerol. The most abundant sphingolipid is sphingomyelin, which has phosphocholine as its head group. Sphingolipids and glycolipids are found in cell membranes (particularly abundant in nervous tissue), but only minor amounts are found in adipose depot fat.

Table 4.2 The alcohols contributing the polar X groups in the major phosphoglycerides

Phosphoglyceride	Alcohol component
phosphatidyl ethanolamine	$HOCH_2CH_2NH_2$
phosphatidyl choline	$HOCH_2CH_2N^+(CH_3)_3$
phosphatidyl serine	$HOCH_2CHNH_2COOH$
phosphatidyl inositol	
phosphatidyl glycerol	$HOCH_2CHOHCH_2OH$
phosphatidyl 3'-O-aminoacyl glycerol	
cardiolipin	

Phosphoglycerides (Fig. 4.1) are diacylglycerols in which the third hydroxyl group of the glycerol backbone is esterified with phosphoric acid which forms a second ester link with an alcohol (e.g. serine, inositol) or more commonly an amino alcohol (e.g. ethanolamine, choline; see Table 4.2). Phospholipids are formed in all cells of the body and are important components of membranes forming a bilayer (Figure 4.2); they also play an important role in the process of blood clotting.

Lipoproteins are formed mainly in the liver and circulation and are a combination of triacylglycerols, phospholipids, cholesterol, and protein. Lipoproteins constitute the main transport form of fat in the blood. This is necessary because triacylglycerols alone are virtually insoluble in water. The presence of a protein coat helps to increase the solubility of the lipid it encases. Lipoproteins in plasma are classified according to their density. High-density lipoproteins (HDL) contain the least amount of cholesterol and appear to act to carry cholesterol away from the walls of arteries for conversion to bile in the liver. Bile is subsequently secreted into the gut and excreted in the faeces. The low-density lipoproteins (LDL) normally transport 60–80% of the total plasma cholesterol and have the greatest affinity for the arterial wall. Deposition of cholesterol in

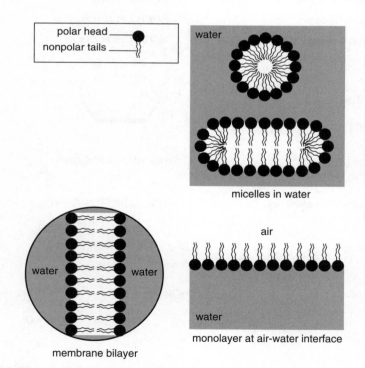

Fig. 4.2 Phospholipid–water interactions.

the arterial wall ultimately causes a proliferation of the underlying smooth muscle, attracts fibroblasts, and promotes coagulation. These changes damage and cause a narrowing of the arterial wall, which in the case of coronary arteries supplying the heart muscle may result in an inadequate supply of oxygen, culminating in an infarct (death and necrosis of a part of the cardiac muscle) which is potentially fatal. The concentrations of HDL and LDL and their ratio in the plasma represent important risk factors in predicting the probability of suffering from coronary heart disease. A high ratio of LDL:HDL increases the risk of contracting the disease. This ratio can be improved (increase in HDL with a fall or no change in LDL) by eating a diet lower in total energy and lower in saturated lipid and cholesterol. Endurance training (regular, moderate aerobic exercise) may also increase the HDL level and favourably affect the LDL:HDL ratio.

Chylomicrons are the largest lipoprotein particles found in blood plasma and contain the highest proportion (approximately 85%) of triacylgycerol. They are derived from dietary sources of triacylglycerol only, are produced by the intestinal epithelia, and are delivered to the circulation via the lymphatic system. The plasma half-life of chylomicrons is less than 1 h in humans and only a few minutes in rats (indicating a rapid rate of uptake by the body tissues). However, the digestion and absorption of dietary lipid in the intestine and the production and secretion of chylomicrons take place for quite a few hours after a meal and hence a lipaemia persists for several hours after a meal containing fat.

Triacylglycerols, whether in the form of chylomicrons or other lipoproteins, are not taken up directly into the cells by any tissue. The triacylglycerol molecules must first be hydrolysed enzymatically outside the cell to fatty acids and glycerol. The fatty acids can then enter the cell; glycerol is transported via the circulation to the liver and kidneys where significant uptake occurs. Other tissues, including muscle, have little enzymatic capacity to utilize glycerol. The extracellular hydrolysis of triacylglycerols is carried out by lipoprotein lipase which is attached to the outer surface of endothelial cells lining the capillaries of tissues such as muscle, adipose tissue, the heart, and lungs. In the liver, lipoprotein lipase is attached to the outer surface of the hepatocytes. Two other enzymes, phospholipase A_2, attached to the capillary endothelium, and lecithin–cholesterol acyltransferase (LCAT) and another lipoprotein, HDL are involved in the degradation of chylomicrons and very low-density lipoproteins (VLDL). Phospholipase A_2 acts on phospholipids present on the surface of the lipoproteins. The enzyme LCAT is present in the plasma and transfers a fatty acid from lecithin (phosphatidylcholine) to unesterified cholesterol on the HDL to form the non-polar acylcholesterol ester. The latter is transferred from the HDL to the chylomicron or VLDL particle as the triacylglycerol is being removed by the action of lipoprotein lipase. This helps to maintain the stability of the lipoprotein particles since the triacylglycerol component becomes progressively depleted during passage through muscle and adipose tissues.

4.2.3 Derived lipids

This class of lipids includes substances derived from simple and compound lipids. Cholesterol (Fig. 4.1) is the most widely recognized and is a sterol found only in animal tissues. Although cholesterol does not contain any fatty acids it does exhibit some of the physical and chemical characteristics of lipid. Cholesterol is present in all cells of the body. It is a constituent of cell membranes and is an essential precursor for the synthesis of vitamin D and steroid hormones such as oestrogen, testosterone, and cortisol. Cholesterol is also required for the synthesis of bile which plays an important role in the emulsification of fats in the digestive tract. The richest source of cholesterol in the diet is egg yolk. Cholesterol is also abundant in meats, shellfish, and dairy products. Cholesterol is not found in plants, and so vegetarians will have a very low cholesterol intake. However, even when an individual consumes a virtually cholesterol-free diet, the rate of endogenous cholesterol synthesis in the liver may be something of the order of 0.5–2.0 g day^{-1}. More can be produced, especially if the diet is high in saturated lipids, which facilitates the synthesis of cholesterol by the liver.

4.3 Lipid synthesis

4.3.1 Fatty acid synthesis

The synthesis of fatty acids occurs in the cytoplasm of liver and adipose tissue cells. The overall reaction is shown below, in which one molecule of acetyl-CoA and seven molecules of malonyl-CoA are condensed to make one molecule of palmitic acid. The reducing power is provided by NADPH:

1 acetyl-CoA + 7 malonyl-CoA + 14NADPH + 14H$^+$ →

$$1 \ CH_3(CH_2)_{14}COOH + 7CO_2 + 8CoA + 14NADP^+ + 6H_2O.$$

In contrast, the breakdown of fatty acids occurs in the mitochondria. The synthetic process takes place by the sequential addition of two-carbon (2-C) units, derived from acetyl-CoA, to the elongating fatty acid carbon chain (Fig. 4.3a). The initial step in fatty acid synthesis is the carboxylation of acetyl-CoA to form malonyl-CoA. This irreversible reaction is catalysed by the enzyme acetyl-CoA carboxylase which utilizes biotin as a co-enzyme acting as the carbon dioxide carrier. The carbon dioxide is derived from bicarbonate, and ATP supplies the energy to drive the reaction in the direction of malonyl-CoA formation.

In the next step, another molecule of acetyl-CoA and the newly formed malonyl-CoA are linked via a sulfide bond to an acyl carrier protein (ACP) by the enzymes acetyl-CoA transcyclase and malony-CoA transcyclase, which are part of an enzyme complex called fatty acid synthetase. The next step is catal-

(a)

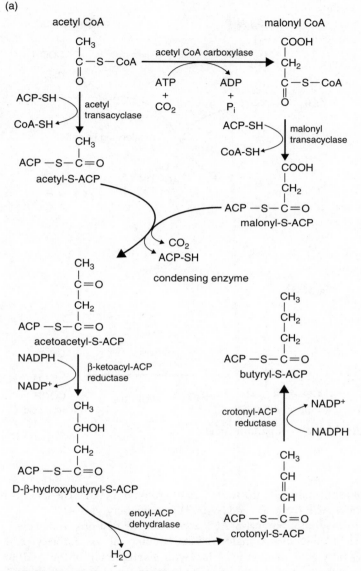

Fig. 4.3a Pathway of fatty acid synthesis.

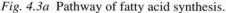

ysed by another part of the enzyme complex: acetyl–malonyl ACP-condensing enzyme condenses the acetyl-*S*-ACP and malonyl-*S*-ACP to form acetoacetyl-*S*-ACP. This is then reduced by β-ketoacyl-ACP reductase, using NADPH as the reducing agent, to form D-β-hydroxybutyryl-*S*-ACP. This is then dehydrated (removal of H_2O) by β-hydroxyacyl dehydratase (also known as enoyl-ACP

(b)

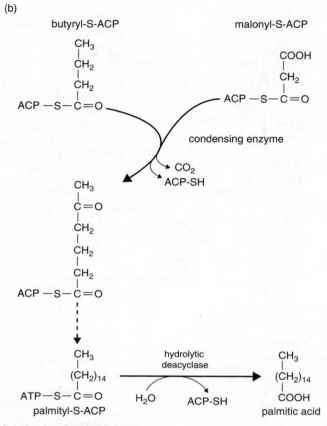

Fig. 4.3b Synthesis of palmitic acid.

dehydratase) resulting in the formation of crotonyl-*S*-ACP. The latter is reduced by crotonyl-ACP reductase and NADPH forming butyryl-*S*-ACP.

The formation of butyryl-*S*-ACP completes the first of seven cycles, in each of which a molecule of malonyl-*S*-ACP enters at the carboxyl end of the growing fatty acyl chain (Fig. 4.3*b*), with displacement of the ACP molecule from the carboxyl group and loss of the distal carboxyl group of malonyl-*S*-ACP as CO_2. Palmityl-*S*-ACP is the final end-product and, at the end of the cycle, free palmitic acid is discharged from ACP by the action of a hydrolytic deacyclase (Fig. 4.3*b*). The overall equation for palmitic acid synthesis is thus:

$$8 \text{ acetyl-CoA} + 14\text{NADPH} + 14\text{H}^+ + 7\text{ATP} + \text{H}_2\text{O} \rightarrow$$
$$1 \text{ palmitic acid} + 8\text{CoA} + 14\text{NADP}^+ + 7\text{ADP} + 7\text{P}_i.$$

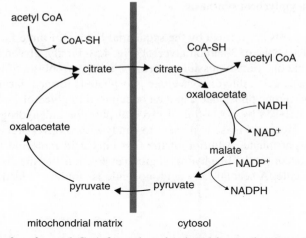

Fig. 4.4 Transfer of acetyl-CoA from the mitochondrion to the cytosol via citrate.

Although fatty acids are synthesized in the cytosol by the fatty acid synthetase complex, the acetyl-CoA required is formed from pyruvate in the mitochondria. However, acetyl-CoA cannot pass directly through the mitochondrial membranes, and so citrate is formed from acetyl-CoA and oxaloacetate in the mitochondrion and then traverses the mitochondrial membranes, acting as a carrier of the 2-C unit (Fig. 4.4). Once in the cytoplasm, acetyl-CoA and oxaloacetate are re-formed from the breakdown of citrate by the ATP-dependent citrate-cleaving enzyme, which catalyses the reaction:

citrate + ATP + CoA → acetyl-CoA + ADP + P_i + oxaloacetate.

Pyruvate is regenerated via the conversion of oxaloacetate to malate and thence to pyruvate. The latter can then return to the mitochondria. Citrate thus serves to carry acetyl groups from the mitochondria to the cytoplasm (acetyl groups can also be carried by carnitine, but this does not appear to be a major pathway). This shuttle process also generates some of the NADPH needed for fatty acid synthesis from cytosolic NADH. The remainder of the NADPH comes from the pentose phosphate pathway in which NADPH is regenerated from NADP when glucose 6-phosphate is oxidized to ribose 5-phosphate. The activity of the pentose phosphate pathway is very high in adipose tissue where large amounts of NADPH are used in the synthesis of fatty acids. In contrast, the activity of this pathway in skeletal muscle is very low. Hence, the fatty acid requirements of muscle are largely met by the uptake of fatty acids released into the circulation from adipose tissue.

4.3.2 Triacylglycerol synthesis

Triacylglycerols are formed by the sequential linking of three fatty acid molecules to a backbone of 3-carbon glycerol (Fig. 4.5). Firstly, glycerol 3-phosphate is formed via one of two possible pathways. In the cytoplasm of both liver and adipose tissue cells, dihydroxyacetone phosphate is formed during glycolysis. Dihydroxyacetone phosphate can then be reduced to glycerol 3-phosphate in a reaction catalysed by NAD-linked glycerol phosphate dehydrogenase. In the liver only, glycerol kinase is present to catalyse the conversion of glycerol to glycerol 3-phosphate. Addition of the first fatty acid molecule from its CoA derivative occurs at the free hydroxyl group at position 1 of the glycerol 3-phosphate molecule. A second fatty acid molecule is similarly added at position 2

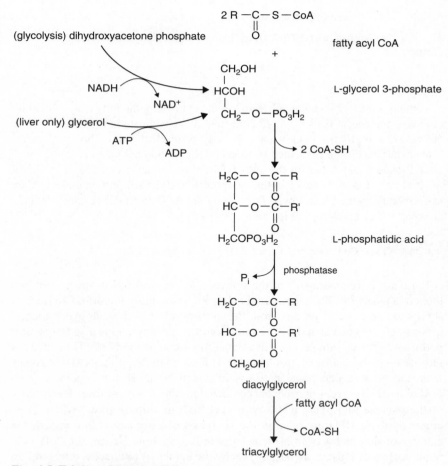

Fig. 4.5 Triglyceride (triacylglycerol) synthesis.

forming 1-phosphatidic acid; both these reactions are catalysed by an acyl transferase. Phosphatidic acids occur in only trace amounts in cells, but they are important intermediates common to the biosynthesis of both triacylglycerols and the phosphoglycerides. To form triacylglycerols, phosphatidic acids undergo hydrolysis by a specific phosphatase enzyme which cleaves the phosphate group from the molecule yielding a diacylglycerol. A third fatty acid is added to this in a similar acyl-transferase catalysed reaction resulting in the formation of a triacylglycerol:

L-phosphatidic acid + H_2O → diacylglycerol + P_i;

fatty acyl CoA + diacylglycerol → triacylglycerol + CoA.

In the cells of the intestinal mucosa, which are very active in synthesizing triacylglycerols during the absorption of fatty acids from the intestine, another type of acylation reaction takes place. Monoacylglycerols formed during intestinal digestion may be acylated directly and do not need to pass through a phosphatidic acid stage:

monoacylglycerol + fatty acyl-CoA → diacylglycerol + CoA.

Triacylglycerols formed in adipose tissue are stored as an anhydrous droplet in the cytoplasm. This may occupy more than 95% of the total volume of the adipocyte. Breakdown of triacylglycerols to supply fatty acids for release into the circulation occurs via a hormone-sensitive lipase (Fig. 4.6). Plasma fatty acids represent an important fuel source for exercising muscle, as described later. Triacylglycerols synthesized in the liver may be combined with cholesterol, phospholipids, and protein to form lipoproteins (HDL and VLDL) which are subsequently released into the circulation and thus made available for uptake

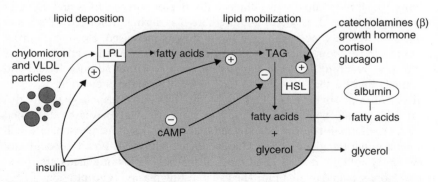

Fig. 4.6 Major pathways of lipid storage and mobilization in human adipose tissue and the influence of hormones. LPL, lipoprotein lipase; TAG, triacylglycerol; HSL, hormone-sensitive lipase; VLDL, very low-density lipoprotein.

in peripheral tissues including muscle. LDL are formed in the circulation when the VLDL are degraded by the action of lipoprotein lipase located in the capillary endothelium. Although the muscle content of triacylglycerol is relatively small compared with adipose tissue and liver cells, the intramuscular triacylglycerol store can be a significant source of fuel for oxidative metabolism during prolonged exercise.

The triacylglycerol stored in adipose tissue and muscle provides most of the FFA that are oxidized during exercise; under normal conditions, plasma triacylglycerols provide only a minor proportion of the FFA. This is because triacylglycerol entry into skeletal muscle is catalysed by LPL, and the activity of this enzyme is not capable of meeting the FFA requirement for muscle during exercise. However, plasma triacylglycerols are important for the replenishment of triacylglycerols that have been utilized from adipose and muscular sources during exercise.

4.4 Lipolysis

Lipid and carbohydrate are the major nutrients that provide energy for muscular contraction. Lipid is principally stored as triacylglycerol. Muscle fibres cannot oxidize triacylglycerols directly; first it must be broken down into its fatty acid and glycerol components. This process is called lipolysis and it begins with the hydrolytic removal of a fatty acid molecule from the glycerol backbone at either position 1 or 3. This step is catalysed by a hormone-sensitive triacylglycerol lipase. A specific lipase for the remaining diacylglycerol removes another fatty acid and another specific lipase removes the last fatty acid from the mono-acylglycerol.

The fatty acids and glycerol derived from lipolysis in adipose tissue are subsequently released into the circulation. Both the rate of lipolysis and the rate of adipose tissue blood flow will influence the rate of entry of FFA and glycerol into the circulation. It is worth nothing here that during prolonged exercise at about 50% $\dot{V}O_2$max, adipose tissue blood flow is increased. However, during intense exercise, sympathetic vasoconstriction results in a fall in adipose tissue blood flow, resulting in the accumulation of FFA within adipose tissue, and effectively limiting the entry of FFA (and glycerol) into the circulation.

Glycerol in plasma can be taken up by the liver and phosphorylated to glycerol 3-phosphate which can be used to form triacylglycerols as described earlier, or, alternatively, can be oxidized to dihydroxyacetone phosphate which can enter either the glycolytic or gluconeogenic pathways. Free fatty acids are very poorly soluble in water, and most of the fatty acids in plasma are transported loosely bound to albumin. The usual resting plasma concentration of FFA is 0.2–0.4 mmol^{-1}. However, during (or shortly after) prolonged exercise the plasma FFA concentration may rise to up to about 2.0 mmol^{-1}. Uptake of FFA by muscle is directly related to the plasma FFA concentration, and hence the lipolytic mobilization of lipid stores is an important step in ensuring an adequate nutrient supply for prolonged muscular work. The long-chain FFAs present in human plasma are mainly oleate (43%), palmitate (24%), stearate (13%), linoleate (10%), and palmitoleate (5%). Their solubility in water is low and their transport in blood is facilitated by the presence of albumin, the most abundant protein in plasma. The normal plasma albumin concentration is about 45 g l^{-1} (approximately 0.7 mmol^{-1}). Each albumin molecule contains three high-affinity binding sites for FFA (and seven other low-affinity binding sites). When the three high-affinity binding sites are full (at a FFA concentration approaching 2.0 mmol^{-1}) the concentration of FFA not bound to albumin increases markedly, forming fatty acid micelles, which are potentially damaging to tissues because of their detergent-like properties.

The hormone-sensitive triacylglycerol lipase in adipose tissue is activated by a cyclic AMP-dependent protein kinase. Binding of adrenaline and glucagon to plasma membrane receptors on adipocytes activates adenylate cyclase and initiates the enzyme cascade that activates the lipase. High plasma levels of insulin and glucose inhibit the activity of the lipase and hence reduce FFA mobilization.

The rate of lipolysis can be estimated from the rate of release of fatty acids or glycerol. However, the rate of appearance of FFA actually represents the net balance between the rate of adipose tissue lipolysis and the rate of FFA re-uptake and re-esterification, and is, therefore, at best only an approximate index of the rate of lipolysis. The rate of lipolysis is better estimated as the rate of release of glycerol which appears in the blood only as a product of lipolysis. After glycerol has been released from adipose tissue it cannot be metabolized by the adipocytes because the enzyme glycerol kinase is not present in adipose tissue. Recently developed techniques using microdialysis probes allow the estimation of lipolytic rates *in situ* by measuring glycerol release into the interstitial fluid of adipose tissue. Microdialysis probes can also be used to deliver hormones or drugs locally to investigate the regulation of lipolysis *in vivo*.

An isoform of the hormone-sensitive lipase is also found in muscle where it functions to break-down intramuscular triacylglycerol stores. The presence of a lipoprotein lipase in the capillary endothelium of peripheral tissues, including muscle, also provides a local increase in the plasma FFA concentration for muscle uptake. The activity of lipoprotein lipase is also increased by a cyclic AMP-dependent protein kinase. The principal substrates for lipoprotein lipase are chylomicrons and VLDL. Hydrolysis of the triacylglycerol contained in these particles reduces their lipid/protein ratio and produces a remnant chylomicron and an intermediate-density lipoprotein (IDL) from chylomicrons and VLDL, respectively. The liver possesses a specific uptake process for the remnant chylomicron and hence most of it is metabolized there. The IDL is mostly metabolized by adipose tissue to form LDL.

Fatty acid transport across the sarcolemmal membrane into the muscle fibre has long been considered to take place by simple passive diffusion. However, recent experimental evidence points to the existence of a carrier-mediated transport mechanism which becomes saturated at high plasma unbound fatty acid concentration (equivalent to about 1.5 mmol^{-1} total fatty acid concentration). In isolated, perfused rat skeletal muscle the maximal velocity of the uptake of palmitate was increased by electrically evoked muscle contractions and was decreased when carbohydrate availability was severely limited, suggesting that certain physiological stimuli may modify the membrane transport kinetics of FFA in muscle. However, FFA uptake into muscle will only occur if the intracellular FFA concentration is less than that in true aqueous solution in the extracellular fluid (i.e. < 10 μmol^{-1}). The low intracellular FFA concentration is probably maintained by the presence of a fatty acid binding protein inside the cell, perhaps similar to the ones found in the absorptive cells of the small intestine and hepatocytes. It also follows that the rate of uptake of FFA into muscle fibres will be proportional to the difference in their concentrations inside and outside the cell, up to a limit when the plasma membrane transport mechanism becomes saturated. After the fatty acids enter the muscle cell, they are converted to a CoA derivative by the action of ATP-linked fatty acyl-CoA synthetase (also known as thiokinase), in preparation for β-oxidation, the major pathway for lipid catabolism. Hence the priming (activation) of each fatty acid molecule requires the utilization of one molecule of ATP:

$$RCOOH + ATP + CoA\text{-}SH \rightarrow R\text{-}C(=O)\text{-}S\text{-}CoA + AMP + PP_i.$$

4.5 Oxidation of fatty acids

The process of β-oxidation occurs in the mitochondria and is the sequential removal of 2-C units from the fatty acid chain in the form of acetyl-CoA which can then enter the tricarboxylic acid (TCA) cycle. Fatty acyl-CoA molecules in the muscle sarcoplasm are transported into the mitochondria via formation of an ester of the fatty acid with carnitine (Fig. 4.7a). The latter is synthesized in the liver and is normally abundant in tissues able to oxidize fatty acids. Concentrations of about 1.0 mM are found in muscle. The enzyme regulating the transport of FFA via carnitine is called carnitine acyltransferase. Two forms of the enzyme exist in muscle: one is located on the outer surface of the membrane (to generate acyl-carnitine) and the other is located on the inner surface of the inner mitochondrial membrane and regenerates the acyl-CoA and free carnitine (Fig. 4.7b). This transport process may be the main rate-limiting step in the utilization of fatty acids for energy production in muscle. Measurement of the activity of the enzyme carnitine palmitoyltransferase provides a useful indication of flux through the FFA oxidation pathway.

At high-exercise intensities (above about 60% $\dot{V}O_2$max) the rate of fatty oxidation cannot provide sufficient ATP for muscle contraction, and, increasingly, ATP is derived from carbohydrate oxidation and anaerobic glycolysis. Energy cannot be derived from lipid via anaerobic pathways. Once released into the

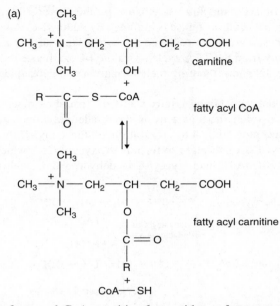

Fig. 4.7a The fatty acyl-CoA–carnitine fatty acid transferase reaction.

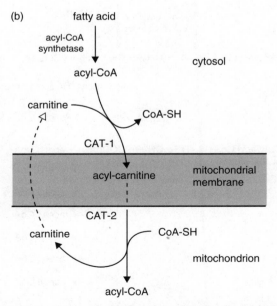

Fig. 4.7b Entry of fatty acids as acyl-CoA into the mitochondrion via acyl-carnitine.

mitochondrial matrix, the fatty acyl-CoA is able to enter the β-oxidation pathway. Carnitine acyltransferase is inhibited by malonyl-CoA, a precursor for fatty acid synthesis. When the ATP supply is sufficient, surplus acetyl-CoA will be diverted away from the TCA cycle to malonyl-CoA, hence reducing catabolism of fatty acids and promoting their formation and subsequent triglyceride synthesis.

Once inside the mitochondria, fatty acyl-CoA is first oxidized to enoyl-CoA by fatty acyl-CoA dehydrogenase using flavin-adenine dinucleotide (FAD) as the electron acceptor (Fig. 4.8). Hydration of the enoyl-CoA subsequently occurs via enoyl-CoA hydratase to form hydroxyacyl-CoA which is then oxidized to ketoacyl-CoA by hydroxyacyl-CoA dehydrogenase. This reaction is the

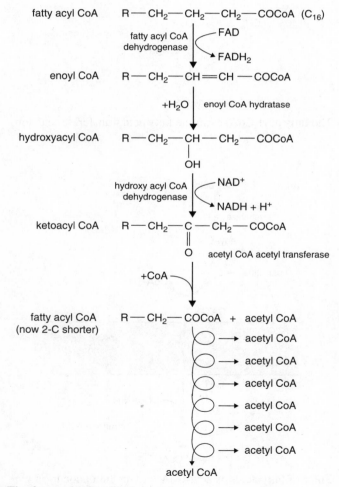

Fig. 4.8 The fatty acid β-oxidation cycle.

rate-limiting step in the β-oxidation pathway. The activity of hydroxyacyl-CoA dehydrogenase is altered in response to dietary manipulation and by exercise; the basis of this control is through substrate availability. The final step in the pathway is catalysed by acetyl-CoA acetyltransferase and results in the cleavage of ketoacyl-CoA, releasing a molecule of acetyl-CoA and a fatty acyl-CoA which is now a 2-C unit shorter. This fatty acyl-CoA can now repeat the cycle, while the acetyl-CoA formed can enter the TCA cycle. It has not been possible to detect intermediates in the pathway, although both acyl-CoA and acetyl-CoA are found in tissues that oxidize fatty acids. Hence, it is probable that the product of one reaction is transferred directly to the enzyme catalysing the next step in the sequence, so that the overall process of β-oxidation can be considered to be catalysed by a multi-enzyme complex. At each passage through the cycle, the fatty acid chain loses a 2-C fragment as acetyl-CoA and two pairs of hydrogen atoms to specific acceptors. The 16-carbon palmitic acid thus undergoes a total of seven such cycles, to yield in total 8 molecules of acetyl-CoA and 14 pairs of hydrogen atoms. The palmitic acid only needs to be primed or activated with CoA once, since at the end of each cycle the shortened fatty acid appears as its CoA ester. The most common fatty acids oxidized contain 16 (e.g. palmitic acid) or 18 (e.g. oleic acid) carbons in the acyl chain.

The 14 pairs of hydrogen atoms removed during β-oxidation of palmitic acid enter the mitochondrial respiratory chain, 7 pairs in the form of the reduced flavin coenzyme of fatty acyl-CoA dehydrogenase and 7 pairs in the form of NADH. The passage of electrons from $FADH_2$ to oxygen and from NADH to oxygen leads to the expected number of oxidative phosphorylations of ADP (namely 2 ATP from each $FADH_2$ and 3 ATP from each NADH). Hence a total of 5 molecules of ATP are formed per molecule of acetyl-CoA cleaved:

$$1 \text{ palmitoyl CoA} + 7\text{CoA} + 7O_2 + 35\text{ADP} + 35P_i \rightarrow$$
$$8 \text{ acetyl CoA} + 35\text{ATP} + 42H_2O.$$

The 8 molecules of acetyl-CoA can enter the TCA cycle, and the following equation represents the balance sheet for their oxidation and the coupled phosphorylations:

$$8 \text{ acetyl-CoA} + 16O_2 + 96\text{ADP} + 96P_i \rightarrow$$
$$8\text{CoA} + 96\text{ATP} + 104H_2O + 16CO_2.$$

Combining the two equations above gives the overall equation:

$$1 \text{ palmitoyl-CoA} + 23O_2 + 131\text{ADP} + 131P_i \rightarrow$$
$$1 \text{ CoA} + 16CO_2 + 146H_2O + 131\text{ATP}.$$

Since one molecule of ATP was required to activate the free fatty acid to begin with, the net yield for the complete oxidation of one molecule of palmitic acid is 130 molecules of ATP.

The oxidation of fatty acids containing an uneven number of carbon atoms in the fatty acyl chain proceeds through the same sequential 2-C cleavage steps as that of fatty acids with an even number of carbons, until the final 3-C moiety (propionyl-CoA) is converted via methylmalonyl-CoA into succinyl-CoA which can then enter the TCA cycle.

The oxidation of unsaturated fatty acids such as oleic acid presents two problems. First, the double bonds of naturally occurring unsaturated fatty acids are in the *cis* geometrical configuration, whereas the $\Delta^{2,3}$-unsaturated acyl-CoA esters functioning as intermediates in the oxidation of saturated fatty acids are *trans*. Second, the double bonds of most unsaturated fatty acids occur at such positions in the carbon chain that successive removal of 2-C fragments from the carboxyl end up to the point of the first double bond yields a $\Delta^{3,4}$-unsaturated fatty acyl-CoA (Fig. 4.9*a*) rather than the $\Delta^{2,3}$-fatty acyl-CoA serving as an intermediate in the fatty acid oxidation cycle. Enoylhydratase cannot hydrate $\Delta^{3,4}$-unsaturated fatty acyl-CoA esters. An additional enzyme in the sequence is required which is $\Delta^{3,4}$-*cis*–$\Delta^{2,3}$-*trans*–enoyl-CoA isomerase which catalyses the reversible shift of the double bond from the $\Delta^{3,4}$-*cis* to the $\Delta^{2,3}$-*trans* configuration (Fig. 4.9*b*). The resulting $\Delta^{2,3}$-*trans* unsaturated fatty acyl-CoA is the normal substrate for the next enzyme in the fatty acid oxidation sequence, enoyl hydratase, which

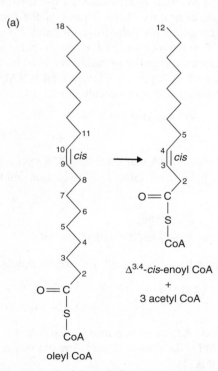

Fig. 4.9a Oxidative removal of three 2-C units (as acetyl-CoA) from oleic acid.

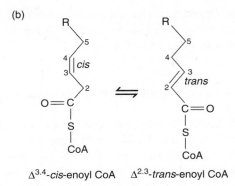

$\Delta^{3,4}$-*cis*-enoyl CoA $\Delta^{2,3}$-*trans*-enoyl CoA

Fig. 4.9b The $\Delta^{3,4}$-*cis*-$\Delta^{2,3}$-*trans*-enoyl CoA isomerase reaction.

hydrates it to form hydroxyacyl-CoA. Hence, the complete oxidation of one molecule of oleic acid by the fatty acid oxidation cycle yields nine molecules of acetyl-CoA. The oxidation of polyunsaturated fatty acids such as linolenic acid requires a second additional enzyme, 3-hydroxyacyl-CoA epimerase.

4.6 Intramuscular triacylglycerol

Although the principal store of lipid in the body is in adipose tissue, some triacylglycerol is also stored in skeletal muscle. Some of this may be contained in adipose cells dispersed among the muscle fibres in the tissue, but there is also evidence from light and electron microscopy for the existence of triacylglycerol droplets located close to the mitochondria within the fibres themselves. Early studies of FFA turnover during exercise using ^{14}C-labelled fatty acids showed that during prolonged exercise, plasma-derived FFA could only account for about 50% of the total amount of fat oxidized, suggesting that intramuscular triacylglycerol could be providing a significant amount of the FFA oxidized during prolonged exercise. Measurements of changes in intramuscular triacylglycerol content before and after exercise lend strong support to this view. Several studies have reported reductions of about 25–35% in triacylglycerol content after 1–2 h of exercise at 55–70% $\dot{V}O_2$max, although more recent work has demonstrated the unreliable nature of triacylglycerol measurement in small biopsy samples of skeletal muscle. It has not yet been established whether triacylglycerol droplets in the fibres or the triacylglycerol of the adipose cells between the fibres, or both, contribute to muscle triacylglycerol depletion during exercise. Human skeletal muscle contains approximately 12 g of triacylglycerol per kg wet weight, and Type I fibres contain more triacylglycerol than Type II fibres. It has been estimated that between 12–20 MJ of chemical energy is available for oxidation following intramuscular lipolysis. The latter is probably mediated by an intracellular lipase similar to the hormone-sensitive lipase of adipose tissue; there is some evidence that catecholamines regulate the mobilization of intramuscular triacylglycerol stores.

4.7 Ketone body formation and oxidation

Acetyl-CoA formed during the β-oxidation of fatty acids will enter the TCA cycle provided that there is enough oxaloacetate present for the formation of citrate. This requires an even balance between lipid and carbohydrate degradation. When the breakdown of lipid predominates and/or oxaloacetate availability is reduced, acetyl-CoA is diverted to the formation of ketones in the liver (under physiological conditions only the liver is able to synthesize ketone bodies). This situation arises during fasting, prolonged exercise, glycogen depletion, and in

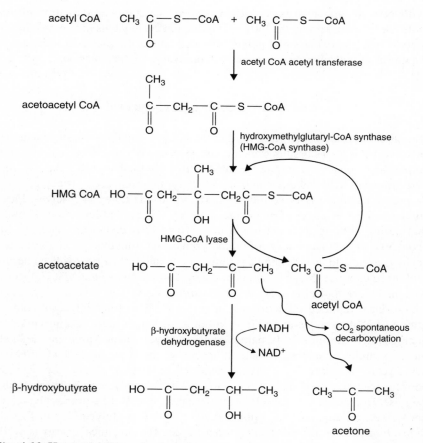

Fig. 4.10 Ketone body synthesis pathway.

diabetes mellitus. Now, two molecules of acetyl-CoA will condense to form ace-toacetate which will subsequently be reduced to 3-hydroxybutyrate (Fig. 4.10) if the NADH:NAD ratio is high in the mitochondria. Alternatively, acetoacetate will undergo slow spontaneous decarboxylation to form acetone. The formation of ace-toacetate, 3-hydroxybutyrate, and acetone occurs mainly in the liver and all three ketones diffuse into the blood. The total concentration of ketone bodies in the plasma of postabsorptive humans is very low, increasing to about 0.1 mmol^{-1} after an overnight fast and up to 3.0 mmol^{-1} after three days without food. Uptake of ketones from the plasma into the myocardium, kidney, and brain provides an alter-native source of fuel for these organs in times of low carbohydrate availability (or starvation) and helps to conserve blood glucose. However, as ketones are acidic, their accumulation in blood cannot be tolerated at high levels. A low renal thresh-old for ketone re-absorption allows significant losses in urine.

Ketone bodies are oxidized in the mitochondria of muscle, heart, brain, and other tissues with significant aerobic capacity. The enzyme 3-hydroxybutyrate dehydrogenase catalyses the oxidation of 3-hydroxybutyrate to acetoacetate by NAD. CoA is transferred from succinyl-CoA (whose main source is the TCA cycle) to form acetoacetyl-CoA by the enzyme 3-oxoacid CoA-transferase. Acetoacetyl-CoA is split to form acetyl-CoA involving the enzyme acetyl-CoA acetyltransferase (the same enzyme that is used in acetoacetyl-CoA synthesis in the liver). The acetyl-CoA formed is then available to enter the TCA cycle.

4.8 The regulation of lipid metabolism during exercise

Activation of the hormone-sensitive lipase in adipose tissue and lipoprotein lipase occurs during exercise due to the actions of adrenaline and glucagon which are released from the adrenal medulla and pancreatic islets, respectively. Fatty acids thus released from triacylglycerols in the fat storage sites are delivered via the circulation to muscle tissue as FFA and from intramuscular lipid depots. These FFA provide a readily usable source of energy that can be liberated through the process of β-oxidation and that can contribute significantly to the energy requirements of exercise. During brief periods of light to moderate exercise, energy is derived in approximately equal amounts from the oxidation of carbohydrate and lipid. If exercise is continued for an hour or more and car-bohydrates become depleted, there is a gradual increase in the quantity of lipid used for energy. In very prolonged exercise, lipid (mainly as FFA) may supply almost 80% of the total energy required. This probably arises because of a small fall in blood glucose concentration and a subsequent increase in glucagon (and decrease in insulin) release from the pancreas. Plasma concentrations of adren-aline and cortisol also increase as exercise progresses. These hormonal changes stimulate the mobilization and subsequent utilization of lipids for energy. The uptake of FFA by working muscle rises during 1–4 h of continuous moderate exercise (Fig. 4.11). The lipolytic process is stimulated by exercise, but this

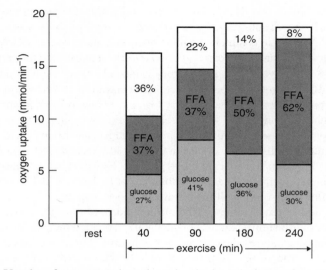

Fig. 4.11 Uptake of oxygen and nutrients by the legs during prolonged moderate-intensity exercise. Shaded areas represent the proportion of total oxygen uptake contributed by the oxidation of FFA and blood glucose. Open areas indicate the oxidation of non-blood-borne (intramuscular) fuels (glycogen, triglyceride, and protein). (From Ahlborg *et al.* 1974.)

process only occurs gradually. Furthermore, it does not cease immediately after exercise has stopped. The circulating FFA concentration reflects the balance between the FFA entry into the circulation (mainly from adipose tissue depots) and the uptake of FFA by various tissues. Although the concentration of FFA in blood plasma is quite low (usually in the range 0.2 to 2.0 mmol^{-1}), their plasma half-life is very short, less than 2 min in fact, indicating a rapid rate of uptake by tissues. At the onset of exercise, muscle capillaries open up hence facilitating FFA uptake, and this process is reversed shortly after the end of exercise. Consequently, plasma FFA concentrations are commonly observed to fall in the early stages of exercise and then gradually increase. At the end of exercise, when muscle uptake falls fairly abruptly but stimulation of lipolysis continues, there is usually a sharp rise in plasma FFA concentration reaching levels of up to 1–2 mmol^{-1}.

In contrast to the limited stores of carbohydrate in the body, lipid stores are abundant and, in terms of the amount available, not limiting to the performance of prolonged exercise. For example, a marathon run of 3–5 h duration would require less than 1 kg of body fat to be catabolized if only fat was oxidized to provide energy. Fat is a more efficient energy source than carbohydrate in terms of the amount of energy released per gram. The complete oxidation of lipid in the body yields 37–39 kJ g^{-1} whereas the energy yield from carbohydrate oxidation is only 15–16 kJ g^{-1}. However, the energy yield per litre of oxygen consumed during fat oxidation is about 8–10% less than for carbohydrate (about 19.5 kJ litre O_2^{-1} for fat compared with 20.9 kJ litre O_2^{-1} for carbohydrate). The main problem associated with the utilization of lipid as a fuel for exercise is not the physical availability of lipid as an energy source, but the rate at which it can be taken up by muscle and oxidized to provide energy. This limitation effectively means that fat oxidation can only supply ATP at a rate sufficient to maintain exercise at an intensity of about 60% V̇O$_2$max. In order to generate ATP to sustain higher exercise intensities, carbohydrate must be utilized. Both the oxidative pathway of carbohydrate utilization and anaerobic glycolysis can supply ATP at a much faster rate than lipid oxidation. During most forms of submaximal exercise, a mixture of lipid and carbohydrate is oxidized to provide energy for muscular contraction. Obviously, the more fat that can be utilized as an energy source the greater will be the sparing of the limited carbohydrate reserves, and exercise can be further prolonged. This has been demonstrated by experiments in which FFA; mobilization was artificially increased just prior to exercise by the intravenous injection of heparin. Heparin has anticoagulant properties but it also activates lipoprotein lipase, hence increasing the conversion of plasma triglycerides into FFA; this causes an elevated plasma FFA concentration at the start of exercise rather than the 30 min or so that it usually takes. This manipulation resulted in a slower rate of muscle glycogen utilization and an increased endurance performance.

Consuming a diet high in fat and low in carbohydrate for prolonged periods has been shown to increase the capacity of muscle to oxidize fat, and hence increase endurance capacity in the rat. There have been suggestions that humans can also adapt by training on a high-fat diet, but the same effect appears not to be observed. Short-term (24–48 h) fasting in the rat, which raises pre-exercise plasma FFA concentration via the actions of increased levels of adrenaline and cortisol, is also associated with glycogen sparing and increased endurance, but this strategy is not effective in humans. This is presumably because, in man, it is impossible for fat oxidation alone to supply ATP at the rate required to maintain exercise intensities above about 60% V̇O$_2$max. Short-term fasting in humans results in a decreased exercise tolerance. Raising the plasma insulin concentration by feeding carbohydrate in the hour before exercise attenuates the rise in plasma FFA during exercise and can be associated with a decrease in endurance performance, presumably because of a higher than normal rate of muscle glycogen utilization. However, several recent studies have failed to confirm that feeding carbohydrate in the hour before exercise is detrimental to performance. Insulin acts mainly by stimulating an intracellular phosphodiesterase, which breaks down cyclic AMP to AMP, thereby preventing the stimulation by cAMP of the hormone-sensitive lipase. Plasma insulin concentration is usually depressed during exercise, with the sympathetic nervous system activation and circulating catecholamines inhibiting the release of insulin. Glucose may also directly inhibit lipolysis and lactate may decrease FFA mobilization by increasing FFA re-esterification in adipose tissue without affecting lipolysis. Some drugs that inhibit the lipolytic process (e.g. β-adrenoreceptor-blockers and nicotinic acid) also reduce the availability of FFA and reduce endurance performance.

4.9 The influence of endurance training on lipid metabolism during exercise

As discussed in more detail in Chapter 8, the principal physiological adaptations to endurance training (e.g. increased capillary density) result in an improved delivery of oxygen and fuel (glucose and FFA) to the working muscles and a greater efficiency of extraction of the available oxygen by the trained muscles. The oxidative enzyme capacity of the muscle fibres may be doubled compared with the sedentary state due to an increase in mitochondrial density. In addition to increases in the activities of enzymes of the electron transport chain there is also an increase in the activity of lipid oxidizing enzymes, including those involved in the β-oxidation of fatty acids. Lipoprotein lipase activity is also increased by training, thus allowing a greater uptake of circulating VLDL for oxidation in muscle. Intramuscular stores of triacylglycerol are also higher in endurance-trained individuals.

Increases in the density of β-adrenoreceptors on adipose-tissue cell surfaces increase the sensitivity of the lipolytic process to catecholamines after training. Plasma insulin levels during exercise are also lower than in the untrained state, and lactate production is lower; both these changes promote lipolysis still further. There is also some evidence that local intramuscular triacylglycerol stores are used to a greater extent after training. Endurance training, therefore, promotes the oxidation of fat by working muscle, which means that the limited carbohydrate stores can be spared. It also means that lipid can be oxidized at higher absolute exercise intensities compared with the untrained state.

4.10 Key points

1. The principal storage form of lipid in the body is triacylglycerol, most of which is located in white adipose tissue. Triacylglycerol stores are also found in liver and muscle and as lipoproteins in blood.

2. Triacylglycerols are formed by the sequential linking of three fatty acid molecules to glycerol. The synthesis of fatty acids from acetyl-CoA requires ATP and NADPH and occurs in the cytoplasm of the cells of the liver and adipose tissue.

3. Muscles cannot oxidize triacylglycerols directly. The triacylglycerol molecule must first be broken down into its fatty acid and glycerol components in the process called lipolysis. The latter is catalysed by a hormone-sensitive lipase

found in adipocytes and muscle fibres. Lipoprotein lipase in the capillary endothelium breaks down plasma triacylglycerols.

4. The principal sources of lipid fuels for exercise are blood-borne FFA derived from adipose tissue and intramuscular triacylglycerol. The uptake of FFA into muscle is a carrier-mediated process which exhibits saturation kinetics.

5. Fatty acids undergo β-oxidation in the mitochondria, yielding acetyl-CoA, NADH, and FADH$_2$. Acetyl-CoA can enter the TCA cycle, and the reduced coenzymes pass their electrons and hydrogen to oxygen via the mitochondrial respiratory chain. Hence utilization of lipid energy requires oxygen.

6. Lipolysis is activated during exercise via the actions of adrenaline and glucagon.

7. Lipid oxidation makes an increasing contribution to ATP regeneration as exercise duration increases. In exercise lasting several hours, lipid may supply almost 80% of the total energy required.

8. Lipid oxidation can only supply ATP at a maximum rate of about 1 mmol s^{-1} kg^{-1} dry material, equivalent to the requirement when exercising at an intensity of about 50–60% $\dot{V}O_2$max. It is impossible for lipid to supply ATP at the rate required at higher exercise intensities. The principal limitation may be the rate of entry of FFA into the mitochondrion.

9. The rate of FFA oxidation in muscle is related to the plasma FFA concentration and blood flow, and is also regulated, in part, by the oxidative capacity of the recruited muscle fibres and the availability of carbohydrate stores.

10. Endurance-training adaptations increase the capacity of muscle to oxidize lipid.

Further reading

Arner, P., Bolinder, J., Eliasson, A., Lundin, A., and Ungerstedt, U. (1988). Microdialysis of adipose tissue and blood for *in vivo* lipolysis studies. *Am. J. Physiol.*, **255**, E737–E742.

Newsholme, E. A. and Leech, A. R. (1983). *Biochemistry for the medical sciences*, pp. 246–300. John Wiley, New York.

Terjung, R. L. and Kaciuba-Uscilko, H. (1986). Lipid metabolism during exercise: influence of training. *Diabetes/Metabolism Rev.*, **2**, 35–51.

Turcotte, L. P., Richter, E. A., and Kiens, B. (1995). Lipid metabolism during exercise. In: *Exercise metabolism* (ed. M. Hargreaves), Human Kinetics, Champaign, IL. pp. 99–130.

Wahrenberg, H., Bolinder, J., and Arner, P. (1991). Adrenergic regulation of lipolysis in human fat cells during exercise. *Eur.J.Clin. Invest.*, **21**, 534–41.

References

Ahlborg, G., Felig, P., Hagenfeldt, L., Hendler, R., and Wahren, J. (1974). Substrate turnover during prolonged exercise in man. *J. Clin. Invest.*, **53**, 1080–90.

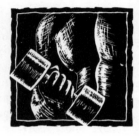

5
Metabolism of protein, amino acids, and related molecules

5.1 Role of proteins

All the genetic information of every species is contained in its DNA structure, and this determines the type and amount of protein synthesized in each cell of the organism. These proteins are, in turn, responsible for the synthesis of all other cellular components: the genetic material codes only for proteins and their component amino acids. Proteins provide the structural basis of all tissues and organs, and it is largely the protein content of these tissues that give them their recognizable shape. More importantly, perhaps, the proteins present in the different tissues confer on each tissue its metabolic capabilities. The presence or absence of a particular enzyme determines whether or not a tissue can carry out a particular function, and the activity determines how fast that process can proceed. Proteins and amino acids also constitute, or act as precursors for, many of the body's hormones, regulatory peptides, and neurotransmitters as well as acting as the receptors for these signalling systems and fulfilling a variety of other functions.

5.2 Amino acids

The metabolism of proteins and amino acids is, in many ways, more complex than that of lipids or carbohydrates. This is, in part, because of the number of different compounds involved. A total of 20 different amino acids are present in the body, either as free amino acids, linked together in short chains to form peptides, or linked in longer, more complex structures to form proteins. All amino acids contain carbon, hydrogen, and oxygen, as do carbohydrates and lipids, but all also contain nitrogen: two of the amino acids also contain sulfur.

The basic structure of all amino acids consists of an amine ($-NH_2$) group and a carboxyl ($-COOH$) group attached to a single carbon atom: also present is an organic side chain, and it is the structure of these different side chains that gives the different amino acids their characteristic structure (Fig. 5.1): at physiological pH, these mostly exist in the ionized form as NH_3^+ and COO^-. The essential amino acids cannot be synthesized by humans, and must be present in the diet, but all others can be synthesized. The individual amino acids, together with the three-letter abbreviations by which they are normally identified, are listed in Table 5.1, and the chemical structures are shown in Fig. 5.2. All amino acids in

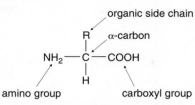

Fig. 5.1 General structure of amino acids, where R is one of 20 possible side chains.

Table 5.1   Amino acids and their abbreviations

Name	Abbreviation	Essential
Alanine	Ala	No
Arginine	Arg	No
Asparagine	Asn	No
Aspartate	Asp	No
Cysteine	Cys	No
Glutamate	Glu	No
Glutamine	Gln	No
Glycine	Gly	No
Histidine	His	No
Isoleucine	Ile	Yes
Leucine	Leu	Yes
Lysine	Lys	Yes
Methionine	Met	Yes
Phenylalanine	Phe	Yes
Proline	Pro	No
Serine	Ser	No
Threonine	Thr	Yes
Tryptophan	Trp	Yes
Tyrosine	Tyr	No
Valine	Val	Yes

animal tissues—with the exception of the simplest (glycine) which is not optically active—occur in the L-enantiomorph form: that is, they are configured such that they rotate polarized light in a particular direction (Fig. 5.3). Optical isomerism and other aspects of chemical structure are defined in Appendix 1. This property, in itself, is of no particular significance, but it does reflect the shape of the molecule, which determines its ability to interact with other molecules. This, in turn, determines the folding of the amino acid chains to form complex protein structures with active sites which can recognize other molecules and act as catalysts.

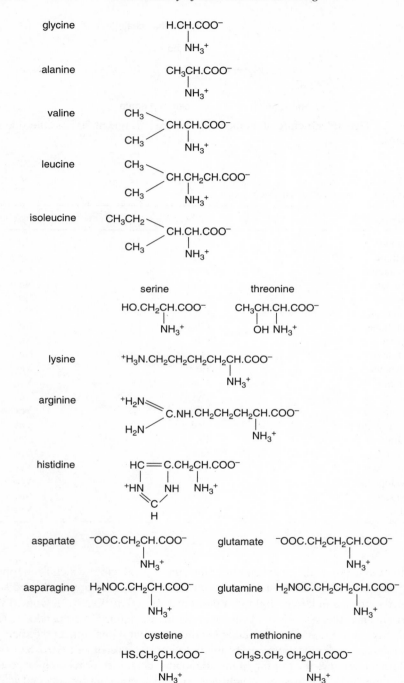

Fig. 5.2 Amino acid structure, with classification according to the structure of the side chain.

phenylalanine   tyrosine

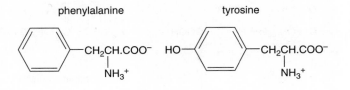

tryptophan

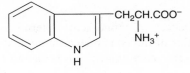

proline

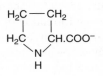

Fig. 5.2 (continued)

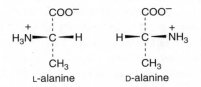

Fig. 5.3 D and L forms of alanine. All amino acids, with the exception of glycine are optically active: the L-form is the biologically important one.

5.3 Protein structure and function

Proteins are formed as a linear sequence of amino acids formed by a series of condensation reactions involving the α-carboxyl and α-amino groups of adjacent amino acids: the resulting chemical bond is known as a peptide bond (Fig. 5.4). Two amino acids form a dipeptide, and longer chains are known as polypeptides. Each polypeptide chain will have a free amino terminal and a free carboxyl terminal. Many proteins consist of more than one polypeptide chain, each of which forms a subunit. The order in which the amino acids occur in a chain is determined during protein synthesis by the sequence of the nucleotide bases in the particular DNA which contains the genetic information relating to

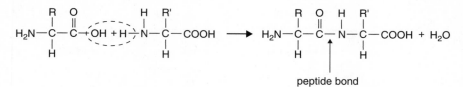

Fig. 5.4 Peptide bonds between amino acids are formed by a condensation reaction. The dipeptide so formed still has one amino terminal and one carboxyl terminal which can make further peptide bonds with other amino acids.

that protein. The sequence of amino acids determines the ultimate structure, because the side chains of the component amino acids attract, repel, or physically interfere with each other, which causes the molecule to fold and assume its ultimate shape.

The primary structure of proteins is defined as the amino acid sequence. The secondary structure is recognized as the result of short-range interactions between adjacent groups which results in the formation of helical or sheet-like structures. The tertiary structure, the compact three-dimensional shape that results from the interaction of the side chains, is what confers catalytic as well as structural properties. Some proteins contain more than one subunit, giving a quaternary structure: haemoglobin, for example, consists of four separate polypeptide chains, two α-chains, and two β-chains. The overall structure allows changes in shape, resulting from the binding of oxygen, to alter the affinity of the other oxygen-binding sites: in this way, the relationship between oxygen partial pressure (pO_2) and oxygen binding assumes a sigmoid rather than a linear shape, greatly increasing the sensitivity to small changes in the local pO_2. The activity of many enzymes is controlled in a similar way, with the binding of regulatory agents, whether activators or inhibitors, changing the shape of the active sites on the enzyme in such a way as to alter the affinity for the substrate.

5.4 Nucleic acids and control of protein synthesis

The development of the cell is determined by the chromosomes which are present in its nucleus, and which contain the genetic information that defines the characteristics of the mature cell by regulating the synthesis of the many thousands of different proteins that give the cell its structural and functional characteristics. The chromosomes consist primarily of deoxyribonucleic acid: the functional unit of DNA—a deoxyribonucleotide—consists of a pentose sugar molecule (deoxyribose), a phosphate group, and an organic base which is either a purine or a pyrimidine. The four different bases which are present in DNA are adenine (A), thymine (T), guanine (G), and cytosine (C). The backbone of the molecule consists of two chains of alternating deoxyribose and phosphate

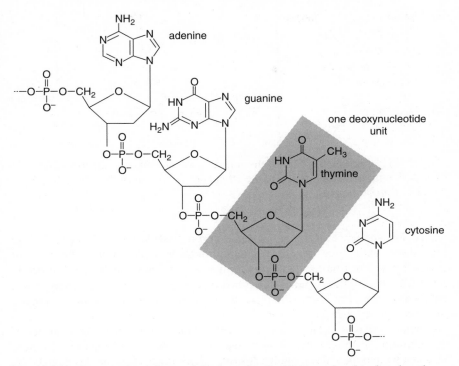

Fig. 5.5 A short section of one of the strands of a DNA molecule, showing the backbone consisting of alternate deoxyribose and phosphate groups and the attachment of the four different bases.

groups, and the DNA molecule is typically tens of millions of these units long: the structure of a short segment of a single chain containing each of the bases is shown in Fig. 5.5. The order of the nucleotide bases in the DNA strand determines the order of the amino acids in the protein which will be synthesized, and the process is switched on and off by control sequences.

The chemistry of the bases in DNA allows bonding to occur between the bases, with strong bonds being formed only between thymine and adenine and between cytosine and guanine (Fig. 5.6), and this accounts for the two parallel strands which effectively run in opposite directions. The hydrogen bonds which are formed are extremely stable, and this accounts for the stability of the genetic information which these molecules contain, but these bonds can be broken during the process of transcription (i.e. when the information they contain is transferred to the protein synthetic apparatus).

During the process of transcription, the hydrogen bonds joining the bases are broken and the enzyme ribonucleic acid (RNA) polymerase forms a sequence of ribonucleotides, following the same base-pairing arrangement as in the DNA strand with the exception of that uracil (U) rather than thymine is present in

permissible pairing

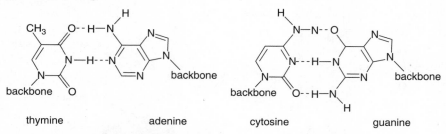

thymine   adenine   cytosine   guanine

Fig. 5.6 The specific bonding of thymine to adenine and cytosine to guanine means that the structure of one of the strands of DNA determines the composition of the other.

RNA. The sequence of the bases in the original DNA molecule (or at least in one strand of it—the other strand is not used—thus determines the order of bases on the RNA molecule, known as messenger RNA (mRNA), as shown in Fig. 5.7. The mRNA is translocated from the nucleus of the cell (where it was formed) to the cytoplasm, which is where the ribosomes (the protein-synthetic machinery) are located.

The process of translation allows the information contained in the sequence of bases on the mRNA molecule to be used to determine the sequence of amino acids in the polypeptide chain that is synthesized. Each amino acid is denoted by a specific sequence of three base pairs—the genetic code—with each of these sequences being known as a codon. Transfer RNA molecules (tRNA) contain one specific binding site (an anticodon) which recognizes and binds to the codon, and another which binds the appropriate amino acid. The amino acids are thus brought into proximity and form peptide bonds in the appropriate sequence (Fig. 5.7). The process is initiated when the first tRNA molecule together with its bound amino acid is positioned on the mRNA: this first amino acid is *always* methionine, and the rate at which this initiation step occurs is probably crucial in the overall control of the rate of protein synthesis. Elongation of the peptide chain is terminated when a sequence of codons which do not correspond to any of the amino acids is encountered.

Each cell in the human body contains all the genetic information necessary to make all the other cells, but this information remains repressed, and it is this partial expression of the genetic information that distinguishes a muscle cell from a kidney cell. The adaptations that occur in muscle with training reflect a change in the expression of the genetic material: endurance training results in an increase in the rate of synthesis of the oxidative enzymes. The control of protein synthesis and the expression of the genetic material can be achieved in a number of different ways.

Transcriptional control alters the concentration of mRNA, and this may be particularly important in the liver where a number of proteins have short half-

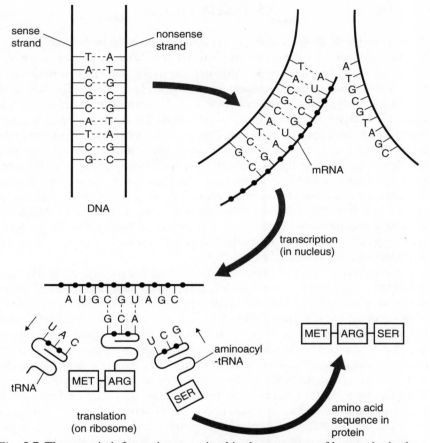

Fig. 5.7 The genetic information contained in the sequence of base pairs in the DNA molecule is transcribed by the messenger RNA molecule under the control of mRNA polymerase. On the ribosome, this information is then translated into a specific sequence of amino acids which are positioned by transfer RNA molecules with the appropriate anticodons.

lives. Control is achieved by the regulation of the activity of the mRNA polymerase: repressor proteins, which are activated or inhibited depending on the availability of specific substrates, allow this control to be exerted.

Translational control occurs at the point of assembly of the amino acids under the control of RNA and without any change in the amount of RNA. There is some uncertainty as to how this control is achieved, but it probably involves the initiation process.

5.5 Protein turnover

There is no mechanism for storing excess dietary proteins in the body, and any amino acids that are ingested in excess of the immediate requirement are oxidized and the nitrogen excreted. Although the overall structure of the body is fairly stable, many of the component tissue proteins have a relatively short lifespan in the body. Most structural proteins and enzymes are synthesized and degraded at high rates, and as much as 20% of the basal rate of energy expenditure is the result of protein turnover. This process is obviously important in the repair of damaged tissue and in wound-healing, but is also an ongoing process in healthy tissue. The half-life of some proteins is extremely short: some enzymes in the liver have a half-life of less than 1 h. Changes in the amount of these enzymes is an important factor in the control of their activity, and a high rate of turnover is, therefore, essential if the tissue is to be responsive to changes in metabolic requirements. In the liver, a high rate of turnover of the enzymes which regulate fuel homeostasis allows regulation to occur rapidly in response to feeding and to short-term fasting.

Some proteins are much more stable, with half-lives measured in days and weeks rather than hours: skeletal muscle adapts to training and detraining with a time-course that can be measured in days, giving some indication of the rate of turnover of the enzymes involved in the process of adaptation. Measurement of the rate of change of the activity of different enzymes shows that some respond quickly: in response to chronic electrical stimulation, an increase in the activity of hexokinase in muscle can be detected within 24 h, and the activity can double within 3 days. Changes in the oxidative enzymes occur more slowly, and peak changes—up to 12-fold increases in the activity of individual enzymes—with electrical stimulation of animal muscle occur after about 2–5 weeks of constant (24 h per day) stimulation. In contrast, physiological parameters, such as the whole-body maximum oxygen uptake, change much more slowly with training and detraining. It is also clear that the changes in maximum oxygen uptake that occur with training are far smaller than the changes in the activity of these enzymes.

Breakdown of proteins into their component amino acids is achieved by hydrolytic enzymes (including a number of different proteinases and peptidases): these are derived from the lysosomes, which can engulf and digest intracellular structures, but they may also exist in soluble form. The mechanisms which control the activity of these enzymes are not well understood, but the process is clearly influenced by insulin, thyroid hormone, and a number of other factors. Protein turnover is a balance between rates of synthesis and degradation, and both these hormones, as well as growth hormone, cortisol, and other hormones also have effects on the rate of protein synthesis. The control of protein turnover is discussed in more detail below.

In response to fasting, there is clearly a net loss of protein from the body, as there is no input of new amino acids and protein degradation and amino acid metabolism continue. The loss of protein which occurs in some tissues in the early stages of starvation allows the component amino acids to be available for oxidation or for gluconeogenesis: it has been estimated that amino acids contribute to the synthesis of about 60 g of glucose per day in the early stages of fasting. Equally important is the availability of the essential amino acids released by tissue breakdown as these can be used to maintain the function of other tissues. Skeletal muscle and the tissues of the gut are major sources of essential amino acids during periods of fasting: these tissues are broken down rapidly in the absence of an adequate dietary protein intake, and adequate function can be maintained even with considerable loss of tissue. If starvation proceeds beyond a few days, the rate of protein breakdown falls rapidly: after 2–3 weeks without food intake, gluconeogenesis from amino acids can provide no more than about 15–20 g of glucose per day.

5.6 Metabolism of amino acids

All the amino acids, except those defined as essential amino acids, can be synthesized in the body, and all can be degraded to simpler compounds. A detailed consideration of the synthetic pathways for the non-essential amino acids is beyond the scope of this book, but there are certain aspects common to several amino acids.

An important starting point for amino acid synthesis involves the TCA cycle intermediate α-ketoglutarate: glutamate dehydrogenase catalyses the formation of glutamate, with the incorporation of ammonia and the simultaneous oxidation of NADH or NADPH (Fig. 5.8). The glutamate dehydrogenase reaction is unusual in that either NAD^+ or $NADP^+$ can act as a hydrogen acceptor in the reaction, and this may play a role in maintaining the balance of the oxidation–

$NH_3 + \alpha$-ketoglutaric acid $+ NADPH + H^+ \longrightarrow$ L-glutamic acid $+ NADP^+$

$NH_3 +$ glutamic acid $+ ATP \longrightarrow$ glutamine $+ ADP + P_i$

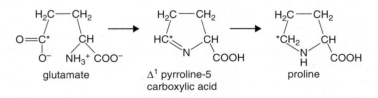

glutamic acid + pyruvic acid $\longrightarrow \alpha$-ketoglutaric acid + alanine

Fig. 5.8 Reactions involved in the synthesis of amino acids, with α-ketoglutarate as a starting point.

reduction status of these nucleotides. The related compounds glutamine and proline are synthesized from glutamate (Fig. 5.8). Other metabolic intermediates can then be used for the synthesis of amino acids, using the amino group of glutamate. Alanine is formed from glutamate and pyruvate in a transamination reaction, and a similar process results in the formation of aspartate from oxaloacetate.

The essential amino acids can act as precursors of the non-essential amino acids, with tyrosine formed by hydroxylation of phenylalanine and cysteine being synthesized from methionine.

Many of the amino acids can be degraded by deamination reactions to give intermediates of the TCA cycle (Fig. 5.9), and this may serve an important function in maintaining the intracellular concentration of these compounds. The deamination reaction results in the formation of a keto-acid from the amino acid: the amino group acceptor is normally α-ketoglutarate, which is converted to glutamate. Glutamate can be regenerated by the action of glutamate dehydrogenase, releasing free ammonia in the process (Fig. 5.10). It is, however, essential to keep the ammonia concentration low, and for this reason, most of the nitrogen

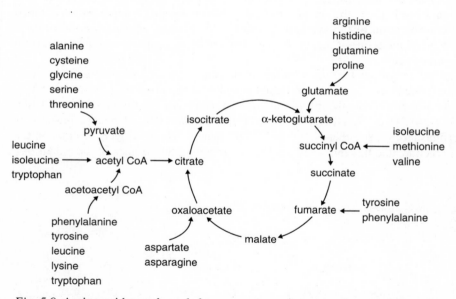

Fig. 5.9 Amino acids are degraded to pyruvate, acetate, or to intermediates of the TCA cycle.

$$\text{L-glutamate} + NAD^+ \longrightarrow \alpha\text{-ketoglutarate} + NH_4^+ + NADH + H^+$$

Fig. 5.10 Deamination of glutamate to form α-ketoglutarate with the liberation of free ammonia is the reverse of the synthetic reaction in Fig. 5.8.

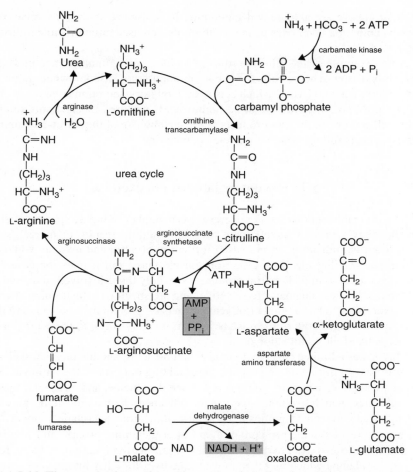

Fig. 5.11 The urea cycle catalyses the conversion of amino groups to urea and thus prevents the potentially harmful effects of an increase in the free ammonia concentration.

which results from amino acid degradation ends up as urea, which is metabolically relatively inert; it is also non-polar and can be excreted by the kidneys without affecting the acid–base balance. The urea cycle (Fig. 5.11) controls the formation of urea: the process is energetically efficient, each turn of the cycle removing two nitrogen atoms but requiring the net input of only one molecule of ATP. Urea excretion in adult man typically amounts to about 30–40 g per day, but may increase 2–3-fold if a high-protein diet is consumed. The reactions of the urea cycle take place in the liver cells. Most of the nitrogen that is destined for excretion from tissues such as muscle is transported to the liver in the form of amino groups rather than as ammonia. The main amino acids released from skeletal muscle are alanine and glutamine. In prolonged intense exercise, the plasma ammonia level rises as the result of an increased ammonia release from the muscle.

As an example of the multiple roles of amino acids, glutamate can undergo decarboxylation in nerve cells to form 4-aminobutyrate, also known as gamma-aminobutyric acid (GABA) which acts as an inhibitory neurotransmitter.

The presence of sulfur in some amino acids requires mechanisms for its removal, and one of the end-products of the metabolism of the sulfur-containing amino acids is sulfate, which is excreted in the urine.

5.7   Protein metabolism in exercise

It is readily apparent that regular exercise has a number of highly specific effects on the body's protein metabolism. Strength training results in increases in muscle mass, indicating an increased formation of actin and myosin, whereas endurance training has little effect on muscle mass, but it does increase the muscle content of mitochondrial proteins, especially those involved in oxidative metabolism. These changes are selective, and are specific to the training stimulus. Exercise also has a number of acute effects on protein metabolism, and the response to a hard bout of exercise is similar, in many ways, to the acute phase response that follows infection or injury.

Muscle has a limited capacity to oxidize amino acids, and mammalian skeletal muscle has been shown to be capable of oxidizing only six of the amino acids: these are alanine, aspartate, glutamate, leucine, isoleucine, and valine. Of these, the last three, which together comprise the branched-chain amino acids, may be quantitatively the most significant. Oxidation of the branched-chain amino acids by muscle results in the problem of disposal of the amino groups, and some of these will be transferred to pyruvate in a transamination reaction, with the formation of alanine which will then move to the liver for entry into the urea cycle (Fig. 5.12).

In resting muscle, amino acid oxidation does not account for more than about 10% of the total ATP turnover, and the fractional contribution decreases during exercise as the rate of oxidation of other fuels increases. Where the availability of other fuels is limited, as in states of glycogen depletion, the contribution of amino acid oxidation to energy provision will again become more important. There are large increases in the oxidation rates of some individual amino acids, and the rate of oxidation of leucine, for example, may increase up to five-fold. This has led to some debate in the literature as isotopically labelled leucine is frequently used as a marker for protein turnover: in situations, such as exercise, where there is a differential effect on leucine oxidation and whole-body protein oxidation, its use in this way is clearly invalid.

In prolonged exercise at moderate intensity, the contribution of protein metabolism to energy production is probably not more than about 6% of the total

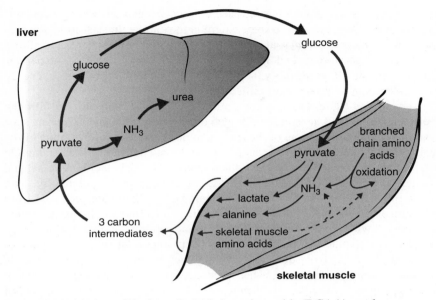

Fig. 5.12 Oxidation of the branched-chain amino acids (BCAA) can be an important energy source for the exercising muscle. The amino groups from these amino acids are transported to the liver for disposal in the urea cycle.

energy demand. In the normal western diet, however, about 12–15% of energy intake is in the form of protein. This suggests that the effect of regular exercise is to increase protein requirements rather less than the requirement for extra energy intake in the form of carbohydrate and fat. Even in strength training, where body-builders are in the habit of consuming large amounts of protein supplements, there is no evidence that the ingestion of amounts of protein in excess of the requirement can stimulate the incorporation of this extra dietary protein into body tissue. These supplements, however, remain popular, and there is also an increasing use of substances (including insulin and β_2 agonists such as clenbuterol) which are known to promote the uptake of amino acids by muscle and their incorporation into proteins.

5.8 Gluconeogenesis and ketogenesis

The carbon skeletons of the amino acids can be used as fuel sources for oxidative metabolism, entering the oxidative pathway at a number of different points. They can also be used for the synthesis of glucose or ketone bodies which can then be used as fuels by other tissues. Amino acids can be classified as glucogenic or ketogenic, depending on their fate: all except leucine and lysine, which are converted to acetyl-CoA, can be used for gluconeogenesis, which occurs primarily in the liver, but also to some extent in the kidney. In starvation, the production of glucose by this route becomes quantitatively important, and allows the large energy store locked up in protein to be made available. Some tissues, such as the gut, are particularly labile, and make major contributions to energy demand even in relatively short-term fasting.

Alanine and glutamine are key amino acids in the transport of nitrogen between tissues, and most of the nitrogen observed to leave muscle during starvation is in the form of one of these two amino acids. This allows some of the energy available in those amino acids that can be catabolized by skeletal muscle (including especially the branched-chain amino acids, leucine, isoleucine, and valine) to be made available for ATP resynthesis, with the potentially toxic ammonia being removed by these two amino acids. Pyruvate produced from glucose or glycogen by glycolysis is readily converted to alanine by transamination, with a number of different amino acids acting as amino group donors. The alanine that is released may be an important substrate for gluconeogenesis in the liver during starvation, but is almost certainly of little significance in the fed state, when gluconeogenesis is suppressed. Even in fasting, however, the glucose–alanine cycle (Fig. 5.13) may be less important than is often thought, since the rate of glycolysis in muscle will be low in resting conditions, and the release of lactate will predominate if the muscle is active. There is evidence for an increased alanine output from active muscle, indicating that some of the pyruvate produced is converted to alanine, but the contribution that this could make to the maintenance of blood glucose is trivial. The main role of the glucose–alanine cycle may be the transport of potentially toxic ammonia from the muscle to the liver for urea formation, thus allowing continued protein degradation, rather than the supply of a gluconeogenic precursor: in this situation, the cycle will be incomplete, as the glucose is more likely to be used by tissues other than muscle, and the pyruvate used in the formation of alanine is probably derived from amino acid oxidation rather than glycolysis.

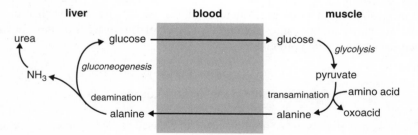

Fig. 5.13 The glucose–alanine cycle can theoretically make the protein content of the muscle available for gluconeogenesis in the liver, but may be more important for the transport of nitrogen out of muscle when protein breakdown and amino acid oxidation are occurring.

The glutamine released from muscle also removes nitrogen, but it may be an important fuel for other tissues, especially the cells in the intestine and those of the immune system: glutamine is known to be the major fuel for oxidative metabolism in these tissues. In the absence of dietary intake, they may be dependent on the skeletal muscles for the provision of this energy substrate. When the demand for glutamine is high, as during periods of trauma or infection, there may be a large loss of glutamine from the muscle, and muscle mass may fall dramatically in these situations.

5.9 Control of protein turnover

The integrated control of protein synthesis and degradation is complex and not well understood, but progress has been made in the understanding of some parts of the overall process. The uncertainties are, in large part, due to the diversity and complexity of the reactions in which the amino acids participate, but are also a reflection of the many factors that influence parts of the whole-body nitrogen balance.

The balance between the anabolic reactions which drive protein synthesis and the catabolic reactions which control protein degradation is disturbed by many factors, of which exercise is one. More dramatic effects are seen, however, in response to conditions such as infection, in which a high rate of protein degradation and nitrogen loss from the body occur. An anabolic state is induced in skeletal muscle in response to weight training, but endurance training has no such effect. Although strength athletes have learned by experience the most effective ways to stimulate muscle hypertrophy, the mechanisms by which these effects are achieved remain unclear.

In the normal adult human, a number of hormones are known to have anabolic effects. Growth hormone is secreted by the pituitary gland under the control of the hypothalamus. Large increases in growth hormone output (or at least in its release into the circulation) have been reported to occur after short-term high-intensity exercise, but the significance is unclear. Growth hormone is known to antagonize some of the actions of insulin, and it also acts on the liver to cause the release of a family of peptides known as somatomedins. These include the insulin-like growth factors (IGF-1 and IGF-2): these peptides have a general anabolic effect similar to that of insulin. It is known that athletes in strength events as well as body-builders have been using injections of human growth hormone, often in combination with insulin, in an attempt to stimulate muscle protein synthesis and hence improved performance. These attempts have been only partially successful as growth hormone is more effective in stimulating the synthesis of collagen, which forms the connective tissue in muscle, rather than promoting increases in the synthesis of the contractile proteins actin and myosin. Improvements in performance are, therefore, rather less than generally anticipated. There are also negative consequences resulting from the administration of growth hormone, including growth of some of the bones of the face, hands, and feet, as well as increasing the predisposition to diabetes.

It is well known that insulin stimulates protein synthesis, but the mechanism by which this is achieved and the specificity of the effect are unclear. Testosterone has an anabolic effect, which is important during the adolescent growth spurt, and abuse of testosterone and related anabolic steroids by athletes indicates the extent to which muscle growth can be stimulated by a combination of training and steroid administration. Neither training nor steroid administration alone appears capable of achieving the degree of hypertrophy that many champion body-builders demonstrate. Again, however, the chronic use of steroids is not without major health risks, and deaths from cardiovascular disease at a young age, as well as from cancers of the liver, are relatively common in those who have used these drugs.

As might be expected from the known antagonism of the actions of glucagon and insulin, an increase in glucagon activity stimulates protein breakdown. High levels of the thyroid hormone triiodothyronine also increase the rate of protein degradation, although low levels also stimulate synthesis. The mechanism of action of these hormones is again unclear. Muscle activity has a powerful effect on the rate of protein degradation, as is readily seen if a muscle is immobilized: within a few days, a dramatic loss of muscle mass occurs.

A summary of some of the factors that influence protein synthesis and degradation is shown in Table 5.2.

5.10 Biologically important amino acids and related compounds

All amino acids are crucial to the structure and function of the proteins and peptides that make up the human body, but several fulfil other vital functions. In particular, the actions of these compounds as neurotransmitters and as hormones allow the integration of the actions of different cells, tissues, and organs.

Table 5.2   Some of the factors known to influence protein synthesis and degradation in skeletal muscle

	Synthesis	Degradation
Activity		Decrease
Insulin	Increase	Decrease
Glucagon		Increase
Glucose		Decrease
Testosterone	Increase	
Glucocorticoids		Increase
Triiodothyronine	Increase	

5.10.1 Neurotransmitter amino acids

Most of the neurotransmitters, which act to communicate between nerve cells or between nerve cells and other cells, are in the form of amino acids or their metabolites. Individual amino acids that have been identified as neurotransmitters include glycine, glutamate, taurine, and aspartate. Related compounds which also act in this way include dopamine, 5-hydroxytryptamine (5HT, also known as serotonin), gamma-aminobutyric acid, histamine, and a number of small peptides: in addition, the most widely distributed excitatory agents adrenaline, noradrenaline, and acetylcholine are derived from amino acids. The synthesis and degradation of these compounds is clearly of vital importance.

Acetylcholine is the primary neurotransmitter linking activity in motor nerves with activation of the contractile machinery in the skeletal muscles. Acetylcholine is synthesized in nerve cells by the transfer of an acetyl group from acetyl-CoA to choline: the choline may be recycled from acetylcholine that has previously been released into the synapse, or it may be synthesized from phosphatidylethanolamine which, in turn, is derived from serine. Deactivation of acetylcholine after its release into the synapse is achieved by hydrolysis under the influence of the enzyme acetylcholinesterase: most of the choline released in this process is taken back up into the presynaptic terminal. During sustained activity, the amount of acetylcholine released in response to depolarization of the presynaptic nerve is known to decrease, but there is no evidence that the availability of acetylcholine in the presynaptic terminal will limit exercise performance under normal conditions. In some forms of muscular weakness (myasthenia gravis), however, a failure of neurotransmission is known to be the cause of the subjective weakness experienced.

The catecholamines adrenaline and noradrenaline are closely related compounds: noradrenaline functions primarily as a neurotransmitter, although some escapes into the circulation and has systemic effects, while adrenaline is released into the circulation by the adrenal medulla to act as a hormone. The catecholamines stimulate glycogenolysis in liver and muscle and also increase the rate of triglyceride hydrolysis in adipose tissue, causing the plasma free fatty-acid concentration to rise. The release of insulin is also blocked by a rise in the plasma catecholamine level.

The catecholamines are synthesized from the amino acid tyrosine, and the intermediate compounds dihydroxyphenylalanine (DOPA) and dopamine are, in themselves, important compounds: the reactions involved in the synthetic pathway are shown in Fig. 5.14. The first step in the degradation of the catecholamines is catalysed by amine oxidase, and a further series of reactions produces the end-products 3-methoxy-4-hydroxymandelic acid (primarily in the peripheral tissues) and 3-methoxy-4-hydroxyphenylglycol (primarily in the central nervous system). Detection of these end-products is often used as a marker for catecholamine turnover. The end-product of dopamine metabolism is homovanillic acid.

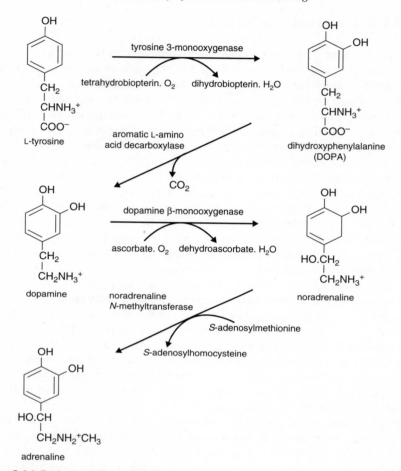

Fig. 5.14 Pathways for the synthesis of dopamine, noradrenaline, and adrenaline from the amino acid tyrosine.

5-Hydroxytryptamine is a neurotransmitter whose importance for a wide variety of functions is now being recognized. It certainly plays a role in some behavioural functions including arousal, and in the control of food (or at least carbohydrate) intake and there is now some evidence for a central component to fatigue which is mediated by the actions of 5-HT.

The reactions involved in 5-HT synthesis from tryptophan are shown in Fig. 5.15, and these appear not to be rate limiting. It is suggested, instead, that the rate of uptake of tryptophan into the brain determines the rate of synthesis, and this, in turn, is controlled by a transporter which also transports other amino acids, including the branched-chain amino acids (BCAA). The ratio of trypto-phan to BCAA in the plasma is, therefore, important, but it further appears that

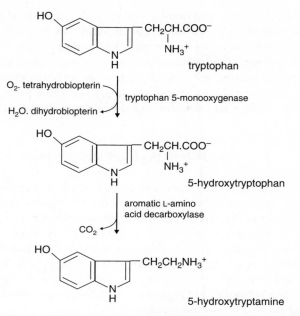

Fig. 5.15 Synthesis of the neurotransmitter 5-HT begins with the amino acid tryptophan.

the binding of tryptophan to albumin is an important factor. Only about 10% of the plasma trytophan is in the free form, and there is some evidence that only this fraction is available for transport into the brain: the remainder is bound to plasma albumin, but it shares a binding site with the fatty acids. An increasing plasma free fatty acid concentration, as typically occurs during prolonged exercise, will, therefore, displace tryptophan from its binding sites on albumin, increasing the free tryptophan concentration. At the same time, there is an increased uptake and oxidation of the BCAA by the exercising muscles, and the circulating BCAA concentration falls. These effects should increase the uptake of tryptophan into the brain, and, in turn, promote the synthesis, and possibly also the release, of 5-HT.

Carbohydrate feeding suppresses fatty acid mobilization, and the low fatty acid concentration in the plasma results in a lower free tryptophan concentration, less tryptophan uptake into the brain and a lower rate of synthesis of 5-HT. This provides for a link between peripheral metabolic events and behaviour. If there is indeed a role for 5-HT in fatigue, this could provide a link between substrate availability and the subjective sensations of tiredness which occur in prolonged exercise. The available evidence, however, is not clear and suggests that even large changes in the circulating concentrations of BCAA and tryptophan may not produce the changes in exercise performance that are predicted if this mechanism is operative.

The related compound melatonin is synthesized in the pineal gland by the further metabolism of 5-HT, and this can act to synchronize a number of physiological functions with changing day length as the seasons change.

Other important neurotransmitters are 4-aminobutyric acid (GABA), which is synthesized from glutamate and generally acts as an inhibitory neurotransmitter. Single amino acid neurotransmitters include glycine and taurine, which both have an inhibitory effect, and aspartate and glutamate which are excitatory.

5.11 Regulatory peptides and proteins

A very large number of protein hormones and small peptide molecules are involved in the regulation of metabolism, the control of protein synthesis and tissue growth, and in the response of the organism to external stimuli. These molecules generally act as hormones, carrying signals from one tissue to another, but they may also have local effects on the tissue where they are produced. The amino acid structure of many of these compounds has now been established, and some have been successfully synthesized. Some of the more important protein hormones and regulatory peptides are described briefly here, but this listing is by no means comprehensive.

5.11.1 Metabolic regulators

A very large number of different agents are involved in the response to changes in substrate availability and demand: the role of some of these and the integration of their actions is poorly understood, and others certainly remain to be identified.

Insulin (consisting of two polypeptide chains—an A chain of 21 amino acids and a B chain of 30 amino acids, with the two chains linked by sulfur bonds—secreted by the β cells of the Islets of Langerhans in the pancreas) and glucagon (29 amino acids, secreted by the α cells) are recognized as playing central roles in the integration of the metabolism of carbohydrates, fats, and amino acids. The balance between these two hormones governs the disposition of nutrients after feeding and regulates substrate mobilization in the postabsorptive period. The primary actions of insulin are anabolic, promoting glycogen storage, reducing lipid mobilization, and stimulating protein synthesis, and the actions of glucagon are generally antagonistic to those of insulin. The importance of insulin is demonstrated in the diabetic subject, when ingestion of carbohydrate results in an uncontrolled elevation of the blood glucose level: this leads to the appearance of glucose in the urine; but it also has other consequences including binding of glucose to some proteins, causing them to lose their functional properties. Excessive levels of free fatty acids in the diabetic person lead to increases in ketone body (β-hydroxybutyrate and acetoacetate) levels which, in turn, results in a metabolic acidosis.

Because the sensitivity of so many tissues to the actions of insulin and glucagon gives these two hormones a major role in the regulation of metabolism, it is hardly surprising that their synthesis and release is tightly regulated. Although their release is responsive to metabolic signals, among which the blood glucose concentration is especially important, a number of small peptides released from the gastrointestinal tract in response to feeding act on the δ cells of the pancreas to stimulate the release of somatostatin, which, in turn, inhibits insulin release. This has the effect of preventing excessive insulin release in response to a rising blood glucose concentration.

5.11.2 Growth factors

An increasing number of small peptide hormones with stimulatory effects on tissue growth are now being identified, but the actions of many of these remain to be clarified. These include the somatomedins, several related species of which have been characterized, the insulin-like growth factors (IGF-1 and IGF-2), as well as a growing number of tissue-specific growth factors.

5.11.3 Gut peptides

Several peptides are released from the stomach and upper part of the small intestine after the ingestion of a meal: these include gastrin, cholecystokinin (CCK), vasoactive intestinal peptide (VIP), bombesin, secretin, and others, including almost certainly a number that have yet to be identified. These peptides play a variety of roles in co-ordinating the response to food intake by regulating the rate of gastric emptying and intestinal motility and by stimulating the secretion of digestive enzymes in response to nutrient intake. There is growing evidence for a role as satiety signals to regulate energy intake. Some of these peptides also have effects on substrate mobilization and storage in the postprandial period, with some of this effect mediated by their role in modulating the secretion of insulin and glucagon from the pancreas.

5.11.4 Brain peptides

A large number of peptides have been found to be present in the brain. As the blood–brain barrier is unlikely to permit the passage of these peptides, it seems probable that they must be synthesized within the central nervous system, and must play some local role, functioning either as neurotransmitters or as modulators of cell responsiveness. Some act as releasing factors, regulating the secretion of hormones that act on peripheral tissues.

The endorphins are a family of peptides that have attracted much interest of late: they appear to have actions on the CNS similar to those of morphine, reducing the response to painful stimuli. The endorphin family of peptides are all derived from a large protein molecule precursor of 134 amino acids, which is split into active fragments ranging in size from the enkephalins (comprising 5 amino acids) to β-lipotropin (93 amino acids). The observation that plasma levels of the enkephalins increase during exercise has led to suggestions that the release of these molecules may be the body's way of increasing resistance to pain or discomfort, and has also been linked to the so-called 'runner's high'. These theories, however, neglect to take account of the fact that the blood–brain barrier does not allow these compounds to cross: enkephalins in the plasma probably come from the gut rather than the brain.

5.12 Key points

1. Proteins, which consist of one or more amino acid sequences, are a major structural component of the body, but they also have functional properties, acting as enzymes and hormones as well as making up the contractile apparatus of muscle.

2. All amino acids have a common structure, consisting of amine and carboxyl groups linked to a single carbon atom. Also present is an organic side chain, and the different side groups give the 20 amino acids their different identities. Some amino acids cannot be synthesized by animal tissues, although they are synthesized by plants, and these amino acids must, therefore, be supplied from the diet.

3. Proteins consist of linear chains of amino acids linked by condensation reactions. Folding of these chains occurs because of interactions between the side groups of the component amino acids. The ultimate shape of the protein molecule, and its ability to change shape, give it its functional characteristics.

4. Synthesis of proteins is controlled by the genetic information contained in deoxyribonucleic acid (DNA). This determines the sequence of amino acids in a protein chain, as well as initiating and terminating the process. Changes in the body's structure and function are brought about by changing the extent to which the genetic potential is expressed.

5. Although the body's structure is stable, there is a continuous process of protein synthesis and degradation: the half-life of individual proteins varies from less than 1 h to several weeks. This determines the rate of adaptation to environmental stimuli, including exercise training.

6. The carbon skeleton of amino acids can be used as a fuel for oxidative metabolism or can be used for the synthesis of other compounds. Proteins are not a major fuel for energy production during exercise, but regular hard exercise will increase the dietary protein requirement.

7. The amino acids alanine and glutamine play a key role in the regulation of tissue concentrations of ammonia, which is potentially toxic, and in the transfer of nitrogen between tissues, as well as in the transport of nitrogen to the liver where it is converted to urea for excretion by the kidney.

8. A number of individual amino acids are neurotransmitter precursors, or function as neurotransmitters themselves. Adrenaline, noradrenaline, acetyl-choline, dopamine, serotonin, and histamine are all derived from amino acids.

9. Short amino-acid chains—peptides—play vital regulatory roles in the control of metabolism.

Further reading

Brooks, G. A. (1987). Amino acid and protein metabolism during exercise and recovery. *Med. Sci. Sports Exerc.*, **19** (5, Suppl.), S150–156.

Davis, J. M. (1995). Central and peripheral factors in fatigue. *J. Sports Sci.*, **13** (Special issue), 49–53.

Dohm, G. L. (1986). Protein as a fuel for endurance exercise. *Exerc. Sport Sci. Rev.*, **1**, 143–73.

Lemon, P. W. R. (1991). Effect of exercise on protein requirements. *J. Sports Sci.*, **9** (Special issue), 53–70.

Wagenmakers, A. J. M., Beckers, E. J., Brouns, F., Kuipers, H., Soeters, P. B., van der Vusse, G. J. *et al.* (1991). Carbohydrate supplementation, glycogen depletion, and amino acid metabolism during exercise. *Am. J. Physiol.*, **260**, E883–890.

Metabolic responses to high-intensity exercise

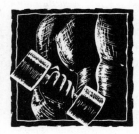

6.1 ATP resynthesis

Adenosine triphosphate (ATP) is the sole fuel that can be used directly by skeletal muscle for contraction. The store of ATP in human skeletal muscle is relatively small (about 24 mmol kg^{-1} dm) and, therefore, must be continually resynthesized from its breakdown products adenosine diphosphate (ADP) and adenosine monophosphate (AMP, see Chapter 2). During submaximal (steady-state) exercise, ATP resynthesis can be adequately achieved by the oxidative combustion of fat and carbohydrate stores. However, during high-intensity (non-steady state) exercise the relatively slow activation and rate of energy delivery of oxidative phosphorylation cannot meet the energy requirements of contraction. In this situation, anaerobic energy delivery is essential for contraction to continue. Typically, oxidative energy delivery requires several minutes to reach a steady state, due principally to the number and complexity of the reactions involved. Once achieved, the maximal rate of ATP production is in the region of approximately 2.5 mmol kg dm^{-1} s^{-1}. On the other hand, anaerobic energy delivery is restricted to the cytosol, its activation is almost instantaneous and it can deliver ATP at a rate in excess of 11 mmol kg dm^{-1} s^{-1}. The downside, however, is that this can be maintained for only a few seconds before beginning to decline. Of course, oxidative and anaerobic ATP resynthesis should not be considered to function independently of one another. Table 1.5 in Chapter 1 demonstrates that as the duration of exercise increases the contribution from anaerobic energy delivery decreases, whilst that from aerobic is seen to increase.

6.2 Substrates for high-intensity exercise

6.2.1 Phosphocreatine

Skeletal muscle contains a relatively large reservoir of phosphocreatine (PCr), amounting to 70–80 mmol kg dm^{-1} at rest. PCr utilization occurs at the immediate onset of contraction to buffer the rapid accumulation of ADP resulting from ATP hydrolysis in the multitude of energy-requiring processes of muscle contraction and relaxation. Indeed, the momentary rise in ADP concentration is the primary stimulus to PCr hydrolysis via the creatine kinase reaction. For each mole of PCr degraded, one mole of ATP is re-synthesized via creatine kinase

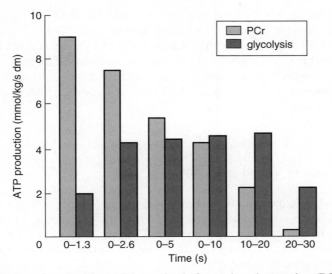

Fig. 6.1 Rates of anaerobic ATP resynthesis from phosphocreatine (PCr), glycolysis and together during 30 s of near maximal-intensity isometric contraction in humans. Values were calculated from metabolite changes measured in biopsy samples obtained during intermittent electrically evoked contraction (1.6 s stimulation at 50 Hz, 1.6 s rest).

(Chapter 2). During the early 1960s, it was thought that the initial 10–15 s of maximal exercise was fuelled almost solely by PCr degradation. This belief arose because PCr is stored in the cytosol in close proximity to the sites of energy utilization, and because PCr hydrolysis does not depend on oxygen availability or necessitate the completion of several metabolic reactions before energy is liberated to fuel ATP resynthesis. Whilst it is now accepted that the anaerobic metabolism of glycogen also makes a significant contribution to ATP resynthesis during the initial seconds of high-intensity exercise, the importance of PCr hydrolysis lies in the extremely rapid rates at which it can resynthesize ATP. This is especially true of maximal short-duration exercise. For example, Fig. 6.1 shows the rate of muscle ATP resynthesis from PCr hydrolysis during 30 s of maximal fatiguing isometric contraction. First, note that PCr utilization is at its highest within 2 s of the initiation of contraction. Second, however, that after only 2.6 s of contraction the ATP yield from PCr is reduced by about 15%, and following 10 s of contraction it is reduced by more than 50%. The contribution of PCr to ATP resynthesis in the last 10 s of a 30s exercise bout is relatively small, amounting to only 2% of the initial yield. The mechanisms responsible for the almost instantaneous decline in the rate of PCr utilization during maximal exercise are at present unknown, but may be related to a local myofibrillar decline in its availability. Considering the high-energy demand of maximal exercise, it is possible that the very rapid rate of PCr utilization at the onset of contraction could be responsible for a rapid depletion of stores at the sites of rapid energy translocation (actomyosin crossbridges). Certainly, this seems plausible because when intense exercise is continued for more than 20 s the cellular store of PCr becomes almost completely depleted, which is likely to be a consequence of mitochondrial ATP production being unable to match the rate of PCr hydrolysis.

6.2.2 Glycogenolysis and glycolysis

Glycogenolysis is the hydrolysis of muscle glycogen to glucose 1-phosphate and glycolysis is the series of reactions involved in the degradation of glucose or glucose 1-phosphate to pyruvate or lactate (Chapter 3). It is clear from the preceding discussion that if maximal exercise is to be continued beyond only a few seconds there must be a marked increase in the contribution from glycogenolysis and glycolysis to ATP resynthesis.

The integrative nature of energy metabolism ensures that the activation of muscle contraction by Ca^{2+} and the accumulation of the products of ATP and PCr hydrolysis (ADP, AMP, IMP, NH_3, and P_i) act as stimulators of glycogenolysis, and in this way guarantee that anaerobic ATP production is maintained, at least in the short term. The control of glycogenolysis during muscle contraction is a highly complex mechanism which can no longer be considered to centre around the degree of transformation of less active glycogen phosphorylase b to the more active a form (Chapter 3). For some time it has been known that glycogenolysis can proceed at a negligible rate, despite almost total transformation of phosphorylase to the a form. Conversely, an increase in the glycogenolytic rate has been observed during circulatory occlusion, despite a relatively low mole fraction of the phosphorylase a form. From this and other related work, it was concluded that P_i accumulation, arising from ATP and PCr hydrolysis, played a key role in the regulation of the glycogenolytic activity of phosphorylase a, and by doing so served as a link between the energy demand of the contraction and the rate of substrate utilization. However, the findings that glycogenolysis can occur within 2 s of the onset of muscle contraction without any significant increase in P_i, and, more recently, that glycogenolysis can proceed at a low rate despite a high phosphorylase a form and P_i concentration, suggests that factors other than the degree of phosphorylase transformation and P_i availability are involved in the regulation of glycogenolysis.

Classically, both IMP and AMP have been associated with the regulation of glycogenolysis during exercise. IMP is thought to exert its effect by increasing the activity of phosphorylase b during contraction (the apparent K_m of phosphorylase b for IMP is about 1.2 mmol l^{-1} intracellular water). AMP has also been shown to increase the activity of phosphorylase b, but it is thought to require an unphysiological accumulation of free AMP to do so (the apparent K_m

of phosphorylase b for AMP is about 1.0 mmol l^{-1} intracellular water). *In vitro* experiments have demonstrated that AMP can bring about a more marked effect on glycogenolysis by increasing the glycogenolytic activity of phosphorylase a. However, because 90% or more of the total cell content of AMP has been suggested to be bound to cell proteins *in vivo*, it has, in the past, been questioned whether the increase in free AMP during contraction is of a sufficient magnitude to affect the kinetics of phosphorylase a. More recent work, however, demonstrates that a small increase in AMP concentration (10 μmol^{-1}) can markedly increase the *in vitro* activity of phosphorylase a. Furthermore, *in vivo* evidence demonstrating a close relationship between muscle ATP turnover and glycogen utilization, suggests that an exercise-induced increase in free AMP and inorganic phosphate may be the key regulators of glycogen degradation during muscle contraction.

Anaerobic glycolysis involves several more steps than PCr hydrolysis, but compared with oxidative phosphorylation is still very rapid. As described in some detail in Chapter 3, the generation of ATP during glycolysis occurs via the phosphorylation of ADP in the second half of the pathway. It was thought for many years that PCr was the sole fuel utilized at the initiation of contraction, with glycogen utilization occurring at the onset of PCr depletion. This is now known not to be the case. As Fig. 6.1 shows, ATP resynthesis from glycolysis during 30 s of maximal fatiguing contraction begins to occur almost immediately at the onset of exercise. Furthermore, unlike PCr hydrolysis, ATP production from glycolysis does not reach its maximal rate until after 5 s of exercise and it is maintained at this high rate for several seconds, such that over 30 s of exercise, the contribution from anaerobic glycolysis to ATP resynthesis is nearly double that from PCr. This is reflected by the very high muscle-lactate concentrations (more than 100 mmol kg dm^{-1}) which are achieved during maximal exercise lasting 30 s or more.

Considerable controversy exists concerning the exact mechanism responsible for lactate accumulation during intense skeletal muscle contraction. The most widely accepted theory attributes this to a high rate of energy demand coupled with an inadequate oxygen supply. In short, when the tissue oxygen supply begins to limit oxidative ATP production, resulting in the accumulation of mitochondrial and cytosolic NADH, flux through glycolysis and a high cytosolic NAD$^+$/NADH ratio are maintained by the reduction of pyruvate to lactate. However, data are available to suggest that the reduction in mitochondrial redox state during contraction is insignificant, thereby indicating that reduced oxygen availability is not the cause of lactate accumulation during contraction. In agreement with this suggestion are data to indicate that it is the activation of the pyruvate dehydrogenase complex (PDH) and the rate of acetyl group production, and not oxygen availability, which primarily regulates lactate production during intense ischaemic muscle contraction. Furthermore, it has also been shown that for any given maximal workload that lactate accumulation can be significantly altered by pre-exercise dietary manipulation This points to substrate and hormonal balance being a determinant of lactate production.

Whatever the mechanism(s) responsible for lactate production during exercise, it is clear that ATP resynthesis via glycolysis cannot be maintained indefinitely. Fig. 6.1 demonstrates that this is especially true during maximal short-duration exercise. The mechanisms responsible for the decline in glycolysis observed during maximal exercise are unclear, but are unlikely to be related to a depletion (local or otherwise) of muscle glycogen stores as levels are still high at the end of maximal exercise. Indeed, it is unlikely that glycogen availability will limit maximal exercise performance until the pre-exercise concentration falls below 100 mmol kg dm^{-1}. A pH-mediated decrease in the activity of phosphorylase and phosphofructokinase (PFK) has been suggested as a possible mechanism which may be responsible for the fall in glycolysis. Phosphofructokinase catalyses the conversion of fructose 6-phosphate to fructose 1,6-bisphosphate and is the rate-limiting step in glycolysis (Chapter 3). However, it is now generally accepted that any potential for a pH-mediated inhibition of glycolysis during maximal exercise is overcome in the *in vivo* situation by the accumulation of the activators of PFK (eg AMP and ammonia). As stated earlier, both AMP and IMP have been associated with the regulation of glycogen degradation during exercise. It has been suggested that once the rate of glycogen utilization has reached its peak, a decrease in the sarcoplasmic concentration of free AMP (as a consequence of a decrease in the rate of ADP formation and/or a pH-induced increase in the activity of AMP deaminase, the enzyme which catalyses the deamination of AMP to IMP) will result in a diminished activation of phosphorylase a, and, thereby, may be responsible for the decline in the rate of glycogenolysis and glycolysis during maximal exercise.

6.3 The integration of phosphocreatine and glycogen utilization during maximal short-duration exercise

As stated earlier, a high rate of ATP resynthesis from PCr and glycogen degradation can only be maintained for short durations. Fig. 6.1 shows the rates of ATP resynthesis from muscle PCr and glycolysis over a period of 30 s of near-maximal isometric contraction in man. The rate of PCr degradation is at its maximum immediately after the initiation of contraction and begins to decline after only 1.3 s. Conversely, the corresponding rate of glycolysis does not peak until after about 5 s of contraction and does not begin to decline until after 20 s of contraction. This suggests that the rapid utilization of PCr may buffer the momentary lag in energy provision from glycolysis, and that the contribution of the latter to ATP resynthesis rises as exercise duration increases and PCr availability declines. This point exemplifies the critical importance of PCr at the onset of contraction. Without this large hydrolysis of PCr, it is likely that muscle force production would be impaired almost instantaneously, which is indeed the case in muscles when the PCr store has been pharmacologically removed or replaced with a Cr analogue. It is also important to note that ultimately there is a progressive decline in the rate of ATP resynthesis from both substrates during this type of exercise. For example, during the last 10 s of exercise depicted in Fig. 6.1, the rate of ATP production from PCr hydrolysis had declined to about 2% of the peak rate. Similarly, the corresponding rate of ATP resynthesis from glycogen hydrolysis had fallen to approximately 40%.

6.4 High-intensity exercise lasting more than 30 s

This chapter is concerned with the metabolic responses to high-intensity exercise (i.e. non-steady-state exercise). So far this has been mainly restricted to examples of maximal exercise, i.e. exercise in which muscle power output declines by about 40% within 30 s of its initiation and where the energy demand of contraction is extremely high and is met principally by anaerobic utilization of PCr and glycogen. However, non-steady-state exercise, albeit less intense, can be sustained for durations in excess of 5 min before fatigue is evident. Under these conditions substrate oxidation can make the most significant contribution to ATP production and, therefore, its importance should not be underestimated.

Table 1.5 in Chapter 1 demonstrates that during 2–3 min of fatiguing exercise, oxidative phosphorylation can contribute as much as 80% of total energy production. This indicates the importance of substrate oxidation during high-intensity exercise, a point which is often overlooked. Under these conditions muscle glycogen is the principal fuel utilized, since muscle glucose uptake is inhibited by glucose 6-phosphate accumulation and adipose tissue lipolysis is inhibited by lactate accumulation. The rate of muscle glycogen utilization during 3–4 min of fatiguing high-intensity exercise is approximately 45 mmol kg dm^{-1} min^{-1} which is considerably lower than the rate of approximately 160 mmol kg dm^{-1} min^{-1} observed during 30 s of maximal sprinting. However, even assuming that only 50% of the glycogen in the former example is oxidized, it can be calculated that the net amount of ATP generated by glycogen oxidation will be about 2 times greater than that generated by anaerobic glycogen degradation to lactate during 30 s of maximal sprinting.

It has been suggested that intramuscular triacylglycerols can contribute to energy production under these conditions, but this seems unlikely given that the decline in free carnitine, which has been reported during high-intensity exercise, would limit mitochondrial fat translocation. The measurement of intramuscular triacylglycerol utilization is fraught with technical problems, and it seems likely that the decline in intramuscular triacylglycerols which has been reported following intense exercise has little physiological significance and occurs in response to a rapid rise in circulating catecholamine levels.

6.5 Repeated bouts of exercise

At the onset of intense muscle contraction, there is a rapid and substantial hydrolysis of PCr and an accumulation of lactate. However, if exercise is repeated over several bouts, interspersed with short rest periods, the rates of muscle PCr hydrolysis and lactate accumulation decline substantially. The progressive fall in PCr utilization is likely to be related to the extent of PCr resynthesis between exercise bouts, i.e. if recovery is insufficient to enable complete PCr resynthesis to occur, this will limit anaerobic ATP resynthesis during a subsequent bout of exercise. However, the mechanism behind the fall in lactate production is less clear. It has been suggested that this response occurs because of feedback inhibition of glycolysis caused by the accumulation of end-products such as hydrogen, lactate, and phosphate ions. However, data are available to demonstrate that the accumulation of several positive modulators of glycolysis occurs during exercise and, therefore, this cannot completely explain the decline in lactate production seen during repeated bouts of contraction. Furthermore, data are available to show that if the recovery interval between exercise bouts is extended, such that muscle metabolite concentrations are substantially diminished, there is still a reduction in lactate accumulation during subsequent exercise. It has recently been suggested that a progressive increase in flux through the PDC over the course of several bouts of exercise may be responsible for this observed decline in lactate accumulation. The authors calculated that the contribution of pyruvate flux through the PDC to total ATP production during three bouts of 30 s maximal exercise interspersed by 4 min of recovery accounted for 29, 33, and 63% of the total energy production. The suggestion of a progressive increase in carbohydrate oxidation over the course of several bouts of exercise is also supported by data showing a gradual increase in oxygen consumption under similar experimental conditions. The decline in lactate production during repeated bouts of maximal exercise also highlights an important point discussed earlier, i.e. that attributing lactate production solely to an inadequate oxygen supply cannot explain the responses observed during repeated bouts of exercise.

6.6 Muscle fibre type responses

The conclusions presented so far have been based on metabolite changes measured in biopsy samples obtained from the quadriceps femoris muscle group. However, it is known that human skeletal muscle is composed of at least two functionally and metabolically different fibre types (as described in Chapter 1). Type I fibres are characterized as being slow contracting, fatigue resistant, having a low power output, and favouring aerobic metabolism for ATP resynthesis during contraction. Conversely, Type II fibres are fast contracting, fatigue rapidly, have a high power output, and favour mainly anaerobic metabolism for ATP resynthesis. Evidence from animal studies performed on muscles composed of predominantly Type I or Type II fibres and from one study performed using bundles of similar human muscle fibre types, suggest that the rapid and marked rise and subsequent decline in maximal power output observed during intense muscle contraction in man may be closely related to activation and rapid fatigue of Type II fibres during contraction.

Fig. 6.2 demonstrates PCr and glycogen degradation in Type I and Type II muscle fibres during maximal exercise under three different experimental condi-

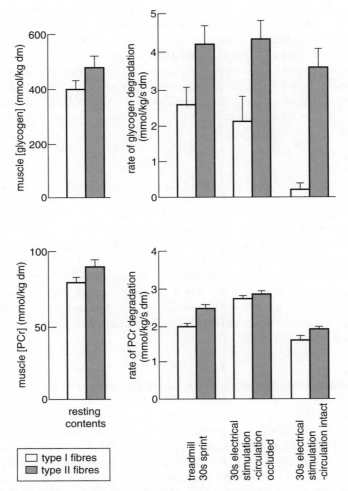

Fig. 6.2 Resting phosphocreatine (PCr) and glycogen contents and rates of degradation in Types I and II muscle fibres during 30 s of maximal treadmill sprinting and 30 s of intermittent electrical stimulation (1.6 s at 50 Hz stimulation, 1.6 s rest) with circulation occluded and intact. .

tions. Notice first, that at rest PCr and glycogen concentrations are higher in Type II muscle fibres compared with Type I fibres, and second, that during intense contraction the rates of glycogenolysis and PCr degradation are higher in Type II compared with Type I fibres. This is true for both dynamic exercise (treadmill sprinting) and electrically induced isometric contractions. The rates of glycogenolysis observed in both fibre types during treadmill sprinting and intermittent isometric contraction with circulation occluded, are in good agreement with the $\dot{V}$max of phosphorylase measured in both fibre types, suggesting that glycogenolysis is occurring at a near-maximal rate during intense exercise. Surprisingly, during intermittent isometric contraction with the circulations intact, when the rest interval between contractions is of the order of 1.6 s, the rate of glycogenolysis in Type I fibres is almost negligible. The corresponding rate in Type II fibres is almost maximal and similar to that seen during contraction with circulatory occlusion. This suggests that, during maximal exercise, glycogenolysis in Type II fibres is invariably occurring at a maximal rate, irrespective of the experimental conditions, while the rate in Type I fibres is probably very much related to cellular oxygen availability and phosphorylation potential.

6.7 Fatigue

Fatigue has been defined as the inability to maintain a given or expected power output and is an inevitable feature of maximal exercise. Typically, the loss of power output or force production is likely to be in the region of 40–60% of the maximum observed during 30 s of all-out exercise. The decline in power output or force loss over longer periods of high-intensity exercise is not as dramatic, but undoubtedly fatigue will develop within 5 min of the onset of exercise. As might be expected, it is likely that fatigue is a complex multifactorial process. If exercise is continued over several bouts, it is likely that fatigue development will become further complicated.

6.7.1 Fatigue associated with disruption of the energy supply

The findings drawn together in this chapter suggest that fatigue, particularly during maximal short-duration exercise, will be caused primarily by a gradual decline in anaerobic ATP production or an increase in ADP accumulation caused by a lack of PCr and a fall in the rate of glycogen hydrolysis. In particular, recent studies have been undertaken in an attempt to relate the decline in whole muscle isometric force production during maximal contraction to the metabolic changes occurring in Type I and Type II muscle fibres. Fig. 6.3*a* shows the rates of PCr utilization in Type I and II fibres between 0–10 s and 10–20 s of electrically evoked maximal muscle contraction. During the first 10 s, the rates of utilization in Type I and II fibres were 3.3 and 5.3 mmol kg dm^{-1} s^{-1}, respectively. However, during the second period of stimulation, the rate of utilization in Type II fibres declined by about 60% to 2.1 mmol kg dm^{-1} s^{-1}, and by the end of contraction the PCr stores were nearly depleted, while the corresponding rate in Type I fibres remained relatively unchanged (2.8 mmol kg dm^{-1} s^{-1}). As already discussed, the rate of whole muscle glycogenolysis does not begin to decline until after about 10 s of intense contraction (Fig. 6.1). Fig. 6.3b shows the rate of single-fibre glycogen degradation during 0–20 s and 20–30 s of contraction. During the initial 20 s, the rate of glycogenolysis in Type II fibres was rapid (6.3 mmol kg dm^{-1} s^{-1}) compared with the negligible rate observed in Type I fibres (0.6 mmol kg dm^{-1} s^{-1}), and was in excess of both the measured and calculated maximal rates of glycogen utilization determined for mixed-fibred muscle. When contraction was maintained for 30 s, as was observed for PCr, the rate of glycogenolysis in Type II fibres declined by about 45% to 3.5 mmol kg dm^{-1} s^{-1}, while the corresponding rate in Type I fibres remained very low. As expected during maximal exercise, whole muscle force production also declined following the initial few seconds of contraction and after 30 s had declined by about 40%. It would, therefore, appear that in parallel with the loss of force production, there was a marked

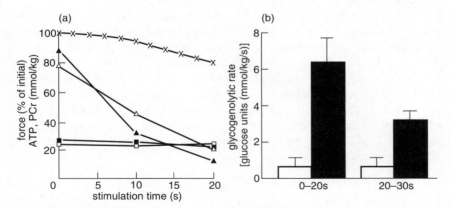

Fig. 6.3 (a) Whole muscle isometric force production (x) and single-fibre PCr (Δ, $\blacktriangle$) and ATP ($\blacksquare$, $\square$), concentrations at rest and after 10 and 20 s of intermittent electrical stimulation at 50 Hz in humans. Open symbols denote Type I fibres and closed symbols denote Type II fibres. (b) Glycogenolytic rates in Types I and II fibres during 20 and 30 s of electrical stimulation at 50 Hz in man. Open bars denote Type I fibres and closed bars denote Type II fibres. (Modified from Soderlund *et al.* 1992.)

decline in the rates of PCr and glycogen utilization in Type II fibres. After 20 s of stimulation, the Type II fibre PCr store was almost totally depleted and the rate of glycogen utilization was beginning to decline. At this point, therefore, it would appear that there is no means whereby Type II fibres can increase their rate of ATP resynthesis/ADP removal to compensate for the failure of these energy pathways. In short, therefore, the declining rate of anaerobic ATP resynthesis/ADP rephosphorylation appears to be insufficient to maintain force production, and fatigue is inevitable. Further support for this suggestion comes, in part, from experiments where repeated bouts of maximal exercise have been performed with short recovery periods between exercise bouts. These studies have shown that a significant relationship exists between the extent of PCr resynthesis between exercise bouts and subsequent exercise performance. Indeed, it has recently been demonstrated that when two bouts of 30 s maximal, isokinetic cycling exercise were performed and were separated by 4 min of recovery, the extent of PCr resynthesis during recovery was positively correlated with work output during the second bout of exercise ($r = 0.8$, $n = 9$, $p < 0.05$). Furthermore, in agreement with the suggestion that the depletion of PCr specifically in Type II muscle fibres may be primarily responsible for fatigue, it was demonstrated that the rate of PCr hydrolysis during the first bout of exercise was 35% greater in Type II fibres compared with Type I fibres. However, during the second bout of exercise the rate of PCr hydrolysis declined by 33% in Type II fibres (Fig. 6.4), which was attributable to the incomplete resynthesis of PCr in this fibre type during recovery. Conversely, PCr resynthesis was almost complete in Type I fibres during recovery from exercise bout 1 and utilization was unchanged in this fibre type during exercise bout 2 (Fig. 6.4).

What is clear from the literature is that glycogen availability *per se* is not usually considered to be responsible for fatigue during high-intensity exercise, providing that the pre-exercise glycogen store is not depleted to below 100 mmol kg dm^{-1}. It is even unlikely that glycogen availability will limit performance during repeated bouts of exercise, due to the decline in glycogenolysis and lactate production that occurs under these conditions. Furthermore, contrary to the account given above, it has been suggested that the decline in the rate of glycolysis, at least during maximal short-duration exercise, is of an insufficient magnitude to account for the decline in muscle force generation that is observed under these conditions.

6.7.2 Fatigue due to product inhibition

As early as the beginning of this century lactic acid accumulation was suggested as being responsible for fatigue development during high-intensity exercise. At physiological pH values, lactic acid almost completely dissociates into its constituent lactate and hydrogen ions, and studies using animal muscle preparations have demonstrated that direct inhibition of force production can be achieved by

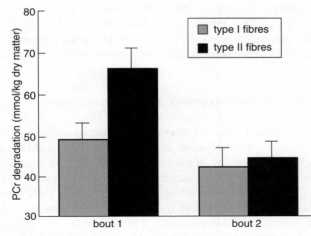

Fig. 6.4 Phosphocreatine (PCr) utilization in Types I and II fibres during two bouts of maximal isokinetic cycling exercise each lasting 30 s. Each bout of exercise was interspersed with 4 min of recovery. (From Casey *et al.* 1996*a*.)

increasing hydrogen and lactate ion concentrations. It would also appear that lactate and hydrogen ion accumulation can result in muscle fatigue independent of one another, but the latter is the more commonly cited mechanism. In support of this, it has been shown that animals which can develop high muscle power outputs or experience severe hypoxia have a high glycolytic capacity and a high muscle buffering capacity. Similarly, sprint athletes have a higher muscle buffering capacity than endurance athletes. It has been suggested that maximal exercise training can increase muscle buffering capacity and thereby offset the deleterious effects of hydrogen ion accumulation during exercise. Similarly, sodium bicarbonate ingestion has been used in an attempt to reduce hydrogen ion accumulation and/or accelerate muscle hydrogen ion efflux during high-intensity exercise. However, although likely to be related to the fatigue process, it is unlikely that both lactate and hydrogen ion accumulation is wholly responsible for the development of muscle fatigue. For example, studies involving human volunteers have demonstrated that muscle force generation following fatiguing exercise can recover rapidly, despite also having a very low muscle pH value. The general consensus at the moment appears to be that the maintenance of force production during high-intensity exercise is pH-dependent, but the initial force generation is more related to PCr availability.

A role for inorganic phosphate (P_i) accumulation in fatigue development was first formulated from work performed using the flight muscle of insects. One of the consequences of rapid PCr hydrolysis during high-intensity exercise is the accumulation of P_i, which has been shown to inhibit muscle excitation – contraction coupling directly. However, the simultaneous depletion of PCr and P_i

accumulation makes it difficult to separate the effect of PCr depletion from P_i accumulation *in vivo*. This problem is further compounded by the parallel increases in hydrogen and lactate ions which occur during high-intensity exercise. All of these metabolites have been independently implicated with muscle fatigue.

6.7.3 Fatigue due to factors preceding crossbridge formation

As described in Chapter 1, calcium release by the sarcoplasmic reticulum as a consequence of muscle depolarization is essential for the activation of muscle excitation – contraction coupling. It has been demonstrated that during fatiguing contractions there is a slowing of calcium transport and progressively smaller calcium transients which has been attributed to a reduction in calcium re-uptake by the sarcoplasmic reticulum and/or increased calcium binding. Strong evidence that a disruption of calcium handling is responsible for fatigue comes from studies showing that the stimulation of sarcoplasmic reticulum calcium release caused by the administration of caffeine to isolated muscle can improve muscle force production, even in the face of a low muscle pH.

It has been demonstrated that when muscle fatigue is induced using electrical stimulation recovery takes significantly more time to occur when low-frequency electrical stimulation is used compared with high-frequency stimulation. This delayed recovery has been attributed to disturbances in excitation–contraction coupling and, as muscle activation *in vivo* is in the low-frequency range, this response could offer some insight into the mechanism of fatigue development.

6.8 Nutrition and maximal exercise performance

It is commonly assumed that nutrition is not of great importance to individuals involved in maximal exercise. Indeed, it would appear that the often quoted need for a high dietary protein intake is unnecessary for maximal exercise performance. This suggestion is based on work demonstrating that the protein requirements of the endurance athlete are in excess of those of the sprint athlete. Furthermore, as stated earlier, it is unlikely that muscle glycogen availability will limit maximal exercise performance until the muscle glycogen concentration falls to unusually low levels. Thus, assuming energy intake is adequate and mainly in the form of carbohydrate, it is unlikely that muscle carbohydrate availability will impair exercise performance.

(A growing body of evidence is becoming available to indicate that dietary creatine (Cr) intake may be a necessary requirement for individuals wishing to optimize their ability to perform high-intensity exercise.)Creatine, or methyl guanidine-acetic acid, is a naturally occurring compound and the total-body creatine pool in man amounts to approximately 120 g, 95% of which is found in muscle. In human skeletal muscle, Cr is present at a concentration of about

125 mmol kg dm^{-1}, approximately 60% of which is in the form of PCr in resting muscle. In normal healthy individuals, muscle Cr degrades irreversibly to creatinine at a rate of approximately 2 g day^{-1}, but it is continually replenished by endogenous Cr synthesis and/or dietary Cr intake, such as meat.

Creatine supplementation is not a new phenomenon. Studies undertaken earlier this century demonstrated that supplementation resulted in whole-body Cr retention, which was greatest at the initiation of supplementation and resulted in a small increase in urinary creatinine excretion. These early studies invariably involved periods of chronic Cr ingestion. However, it is now known that ingesting 20 g of Cr each day (in 4 × 5 g doses) for 5 days can lead to more than a 20% increase in muscle total Cr concentration, 20% of which is in the form of PCr (Fig. 6.5). It is also clear that the majority of muscle Cr uptake occurs during the initial days of supplementation, thus confirming earlier studies. Furthermore, when submaximal exercise is performed during the period of supplementation, muscle Cr uptake appears to be increased by a further 10%. The exact mechanisms by which muscle Cr uptake is achieved and regulated are presently unclear, but uptake is known to be sodium-dependant. Human muscle appears to have an upper limit of 145–160 mmol kg dm^{-1}, and individuals with lower concentrations appear to achieve the most pronounced increases with ingestion.

(Ingesting Cr for 5 days (20 g day^{-1}) has been shown to significantly increase the amount of work that can be performed by healthy normal volunteers during repeated bouts of maximal exercise.)This conclusion is based upon the results from laboratory studies which involved repeated bouts of maximal dynamic and

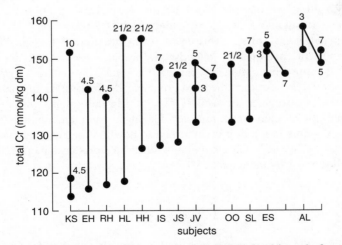

Fig. 6.5 Muscle total-creatine (Cr) content in individual subjects before, during, and after ingesting creatine monohydrate at a rate of 20–30 g day^{-1} for 3–21 days. 21/2 indicates subjects who ingested creatine on alternate days for 21 days. (From Harris *et al.* 1992.)

isokinetic cycling exercise (for example, three bouts of maximal cycling exercise interspersed with 4 min recovery) and from controlled 'field' experiments undertaken by athletes (for example, 4×300 m running interspersed with 4 min recovery). The consistent finding from these studies is that Cr ingestion significantly increased exercise performance by sustaining force or work output during exercise, such that total work production during exercise increased by about 5–7%. The exact mechanisms by which performance is improved are unclear. However, the improvement is unlikely to be solely a consequence of an increase in pre-exercise PCr availability, as the magnitude of this increase (approximately 8 mmol kg dm^{-1}) seems to be insufficient to produce the improvements reported. The improvement in performance may also be related to a stimulatory effect of Cr ingestion on PCr resynthesis during exercise and recovery. Considering that PCr availability is thought to limit exercise performance during maximal exercise, all of these effects would increase muscle contractile capability by maintaining anaerobic ATP turnover during exercise. This suggestion is supported by findings which have shown that Cr supplementation can reduce plasma ammonia and hypoxanthine accumulation and the magnitude of muscle ATP degradation during maximal exercise whilst at the same time increasing work output.

Considering recovery from high-intensity exercise, it is known that individuals who demonstrate more than a 25% increase in muscle total-Cr (TCr) concentration as a result of Cr supplementation can expect to experience an accelerated rate of PCr resynthesis during recovery (Fig. 6.6). It is likely that this occurs as a result of Cr ingestion maintaining the muscle free-Cr concentration higher than the K_m of mitochondrial creatine kinase (CK) for Cr (about 60 mmol kg dm^{-1}) throughout recovery, thereby sustaining a high flux through the CK reaction in favour of PCr resynthesis and ADP formation.

Significant points often overlooked when attempting to use Cr supplementation to improve maximal exercise performance are first, that not everyone responds to supplementation, i.e. muscle Cr uptake is relatively low in about 30% of individuals. Second, the most pronaunced effects of Cr supplementation on exercise performance are usually observed in individuals who experience more than a 25% increase in muscle TCr during supplementation (Fig. 6.7). With these points in mind, it is important to note that recent work has demonstrated that Cr ingested in combination with carbohydrate can increase Cr retention in all subjects by more than 25%.

6.9 Key points

1. ATP is the only fuel that can be used directly for skeletal muscle force generation. There is sufficient ATP available to fuel about 2 s of maximal-intensity exercise and, therefore, for muscle force generation to continue it must be resynthesized very rapidly from ADP. During high-intensity exercise, the

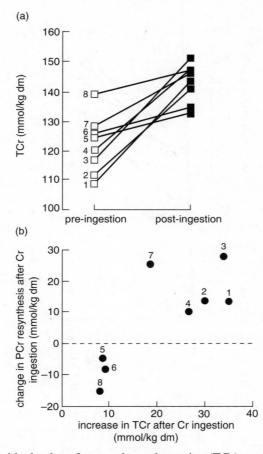

Fig. 6.6 (a) Individual values for muscle total-creatine (TCr) concentration before and after 5 days of creatine (Cr) ingestion (4×5 g day^{-1}). Subjects have been numbered 1–8, based on their initial muscle TCr content. (b) Individual increases in muscle TCr content after Cr ingestion for the same subjects depicted in (a), plotted against the change in phosphocreatine (PCr) resynthesis during recovery after Cr ingestion. (From Greenhaff *et al.* 1994.)

relatively low rate of ATP resynthesis from oxidative phosphorylation results in the rapid activation of anaerobic energy production from PCr and glycogen hydrolysis.

2. Phosphocreatine hydrolysis is initiated at the immediate onset of contraction to buffer the rapid accumulation of ADP resulting from ATP hydrolysis. However, the rate of PCr hydrolysis begins to decline after only a few seconds of maximal force generation. The importance of PCr to muscle energy pro-

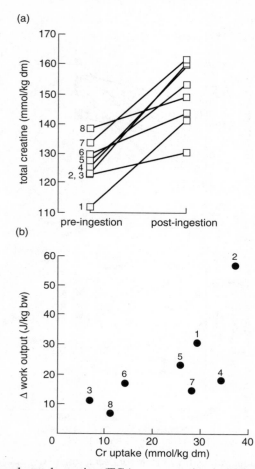

(a)

(b)

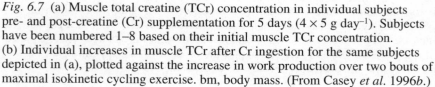

Fig. 6.7 (a) Muscle total creatine (TCr) concentration in individual subjects pre- and post-creatine (Cr) supplementation for 5 days (4 × 5 g day⁻¹). Subjects have been numbered 1–8 based on their initial muscle TCr concentration. (b) Individual increases in muscle TCr after Cr ingestion for the same subjects depicted in (a), plotted against the increase in work production over two bouts of maximal isokinetic cycling exercise. bm, body mass. (From Casey *et al.* 1996*b.*)

duction and function lies in the extremely rapid rates at which it can resynthesize ATP.

3. Glycogenolysis is the hydrolysis of glycogen to glucose 1-phosphate. Glycolysis is the series of reactions involved in the conversion of glucose or glucose 1-phosphate to pyruvate of lactate. If high-intensity exercise is to continue beyond only a few seconds there must be marked increases in the contributions from glycogenolysis and glycolysis to ATP resynthesis.

4. The close relationship between muscle anaerobic ATP turnover and glycogen utilization suggests that a rapid increase in the concentrations of free AMP and inorganic phosphate may be the key regulators of muscle glycogenolysis during muscle force generation.

5. Anaerobic glycolysis involves several more steps than PCr hydrolysis; however, compared with oxidative phosphorylation it is still very rapid. It is initiated at the onset of contraction, but, unlike PCr hydrolysis, does not reach a maximal rate until after 5 s of exercise and can be maintained at this level for several seconds during maximal muscle force generation. The mechanism(s) responsible for the eventual decline in glycolysis during maximal exercise have not been resolved.

6. Submaximal, high-intensity (non-steady state) exercise can be sustained for durations approaching 5 min before fatigue is evident. Under these conditions carbohydrate oxidation can make a significant contribution to ATP production, but its relative importance is often underestimated.

7. When repeated bouts of maximal exercise are performed, the rates of muscle PCr hydrolysis and lactate accumulation decline. In the case of PCr, this response is thought to occur because of incomplete PCr resynthesis occurring during recovery between exercise bouts. However, the mechanism(s) responsible for the fall in lactate accumulation is unclear.

8. Fatigue is an inevitable feature of high-intensity exercise, and it can be defined as the inability to maintain a given or expected power output or force. The onset of muscle fatigue has been associated with the disruption of energy supply, product inhibition, and factors preceding crossbridge formation. It is likely to be a multifactoral process.

9. It is commonly accepted that nutrition is not of great importance to individuals involved in high-intensity exercise. However, there is a growing body of evidence to indicate that dietary creatine intake may be a necessary requirement for individuals wishing to optimize their performance during high-intensity exercise. Also, high-protein, low-carbohydrate diets appear to impair high-intensity exercise performance.

Further reading

Balsom, P. D., Ekblom, B., Soderlund, K., *et al.* (1993). Creatine supplementation and dynamic high-intensity intermittent exercise. *Scand. J. Med. Sci. Sports*, **3**, 143–9.

Bangsbo, J., Graham, T. E., Kiens, B., and Saltin, B. (1992). Elevated muscle glycogen and anaerobic energy production during exhaustive exercise in man. *J. Physiol.*, **451**, 205–27.

Birch, R., Noble, D., and Greenhaff, P. L. (1994). The influence of dietary creatine supplementation on performance during repeated bouts of maximal isokinetic cycling in man. *Eur. J. Appl. Physiol.*, **69**, 268–70.

Bogdanis, G. C., Nevill, M. E., Boobis, L. H., and Lakomy, H. K. A. (1996). Contribution of phosphocreatine and aerobic metabolism to energy supply during repeated sprint exercise. *J. Appl. Physiol.*, **80**, 876–84.

Casey, A., Short, A. H., Curtis, S., and Greenhaff, P. L. (1996). The effect of glycogen availability on power output and the metabolic response to repeated bouts of maximal isokinetic exercise in man. *Eur. J. Appl. Physiol.*, **72**, 249–55.

Chasiotis, D., Sahlin, K., and Hultman, E. (1983). Regulation of glycogenolysis in human muscle in response to epinephrine infusion. *J. Appl. Physiol.*, **54**, 45–50.

Green, A. L., Simpson, E. J., Littlewood, J. J., Macdonald, I. A., and Greenhaff, P. L. (1996). Carbohydrate ingestion augments creatine retention during creatine feeding in humans. *Acta Physiol. Scand.* **158**, 195–202.

Green, H. J. (1986). Muscle power: fibre type recruitment, metabolism and fatigue. In: *Human muscle power*. (ed. N. L. Jones, N. McCartney, and A. J. McComas), pp. 65–79. Human Kinetics, Champaign, IL.

Greenhaff, P. L., Ren, J.-M., Soderlund, K., and Hultman, E. (1991). Energy metabolism in single human muscle fibres during contraction without and with epinephrine infusion. *Am. J. Physiol.*, **260**, E713–E718.

Greenhaff, P. L., Casey, A., Short, A. H., Harris, R. C., Soderlund, K., and Hultman, E. (1993). Influence of oral creatine supplementation on muscle torque during repeated bouts of maximal voluntary exercise in man. *Clin. Sci.*, **84**, 565–71.

Greenhaff, P. L., Soderlund, K., Ren, J.-M., and Hultman, E. (1993). Energy metabolism in single human muscle fibres during intermittent contraction with occluded circulation. *J. Physiol.*, **460**, 443–53.

Greenhaff, P. L., Nevill, M. E., Soderlund, K., *et al* (1994). The metabolic responses of human type I and II muscle fibres during maximal treadmill sprinting. *J. Physiol.*, **478**, 149–55.

Hultman, E. and Sjoholm, H. (1983). Substrate availability. In: *Biochemistry of exercise* (ed. H. G. Knuttgen, H. G. Vogel, and J. A. Poortmans), pp. 63–75. Human Kinetics, Champaign, IL.

Medbo, J. I. and Tabata, I. (1989). Relative importance of aerobic and anaerobic energy release during short-lasting exhausting bicycle exercise. *J. Appl. Physiol.*, **67**, 1881–6.

Putman, C. T., Jones, N. L., Lands, L. C., *et al.* (1995). Skeletal muscle pyruvate ..dehydrogenase activity during maximal exercise in humans. *Am. J. Physiol.* **269**, E458–E468.

Ren, J. M. and Hultman, E. (1989). Regulation of glycogenolysis in human skeletal muscle. *J. Appl. Physiol.*, **67**, 2243–8.

Sahlin, K., Gorski, J., and Edstrom, L. (1990). Influence of ATP turnover and metabolite changes on IMP formation and glycolysis in rat skeletal muscle. *Am. J. Physiol.*, **259**, C409–C412.

Timmons, J. A., Poucher, S. M., Constantin–Teodosiu, D., *et al.* (1996). Increased acetyl group availability enhances contractile function of canine skeletal muscle during ischemia. *J. Clin. Invest.*, **97**, 879–83.

Walker, J. B. (1979). Creatine: biosynthesis, regulation and function. *Adv. Enzymol. Relat. Areas. Mol. Med.*, **50**, 177–242.

References

Casey, A., Howell, S., Constantin-Teodosiu, D., Hultman, E., and Greenhaff, P. L. (1996*a*). The metabolic responses of type I and II muscle fibre during repeated bouts of maximal exercise in man. *Am. J. Physiol.*, **271**, E38–E43.

Casey, A., Howell, S., Constantin-Teodosiu, D., Hultman, E., and Greenhaff, P.L. (1996*b*). Effect of creatine supplementation on muscle metabolism and exercise performance. *Am. J. Physiol.*, **271**, E31–E37.

Greenhaff, P. L., Bodin, K., Soderlund, K., and Hultman, E. (1994). The effect of oral creatine supplementation on skeletal muscle phosphocreatine resynthesis. *Am. J. Physiol.*, **266**, E725–E730.

Harris, R. C., Soderlund, K., and Hultman, E. (1992). Elevation of creatine in resting and exercised muscle of normal subjects by creatine supplementation. *Clin. Sci.*, **83**, 367–74.

Soderlund, K., Greenhaff, P. L., and Hultman, E. (1992). Energy metabolism in type I and type II human muscle fibres during short term electrical stimulation at different frequencies. *Acta Physiol. Scand.*, **144**, 15–22.

7
Metabolic responses to prolonged exercise

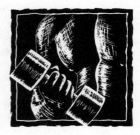

7.1 Fuels for prolonged exercise

The term 'prolonged exercise' is typically used to define exercise intensities which can be sustained for durations falling between 30 and 180 min. In practice, this is usually exercise intensities between 60 and 85% of maximal oxygen consumption. Continuous exercise of any longer duration (i.e. an intensity less than 60% of maximal oxygen consumption) is probably not limited by muscle substrate availability and, providing adequate hydration is maintained, can probably be sustained for several hours or even days. Unlike maximal-intensity exercise, the rate of muscle ATP production required during prolonged exercise is relatively low (less than 2.5 mmol kg dm^{-1} s^{-1} and, therefore, phosphocreatine, carbohydrate, and fat can all contribute to ATP resynthesis. However, CHO is, without question, the most important fuel source during this type of exercise. The major benefit of CHO oxidation, which is often overlooked, is that, per unit of oxygen utilized, it will provide the greatest amount of ATP compared with the oxidation of any other substrate.

At the onset of prolonged exercise, the rates of PCr degradation and lactate production have been shown to be linearly related to the exercise intensity. During this period, PCr and anaerobic glycolysis make significant contributions to muscle ATP production, which has generally been attributed to a lag in muscle blood flow and oxygen extraction relative to the increase in energy demand. However, recent evidence suggests that this response may also be attributable to a lag in substrate oxidation. Without this rapid rate of energy delivery from PCr hydrolysis and anaerobic glycolysis, energy production at the onset of exercise would be compromised. However, following the initial few minutes of exercise their contribution becomes negligible and a steady state of energy demand and energy delivery is achieved. Under steady-state conditions, the oxidation of CHO and fat become the mainstay of energy delivery.

Based upon a maximum oxygen consumption of 3–4 litres min^{-1}, it can be calculated that the maximum rate of ATP production from CHO oxidation will be about 2.0–2.8 mmol kg dm^{-1} s^{-1} and, therefore, it can be seen that CHO could meet the energy requirements of prolonged exercise. However, under normal conditions, the muscle store of CHO (in the form of glycogen) is in the region of 350 mmol kg dm^{-1} and, therefore, alone could only sustain in the region of 80 min of exercise (4 litres of oxygen will oxidize 0.03 moles of glucosyl units, generating 1.15 moles of ATP).

Of course, CHO is also delivered to skeletal muscle from hepatic stores in the form of blood glucose, and this can generate ATP at a maximum rate of about 1 mmol kg dm^{-1} s^{-1}. Assuming exercise is undertaken following food ingestion, rather than in the fasted state, it can be calculated that hepatic glycogen stores could fuel in the region of 45 min of exercise if it was the sole fuel utilized and was oxidized at a maximal rate. However, one should note that hepatic glucose production could supply fuel at most at about 45% of the maximal rate of carbohydrate oxidation and, therefore, could not sustain exercise of an intense nature. Of course, as indicated in Chapter 4, fat constitutes the largest energy reserve in man, but, unfortunately, it also exhibits a low maximal rate of oxidation relative to muscle glycogen oxidation (about 1 mmol ATP kg dm^{-1} s^{-1}). The factors responsible for limiting the rate of fat oxidation during exercise are presently unclear, but obviously the limiting step must precede acetyl-CoA formation because from this point fat and carbohydrate share the same fate. The integration of fat and CHO oxidation by skeletal muscle will be discussed in greater detail later.

It is important to note that the simultaneous utilization of fat and hepatic glycogen stores become increasingly important to maintaining muscle ATP production as exercise progresses and the muscle glycogen stores become depleted. In theory, the maximum rate of muscle ATP production from fat and blood glucose oxidation would be about 2 mmol kg dm^{-1} s^{-1} which is only about 30% lower than the maximum rate of muscle ATP production from muscle glycogen oxidation.

7.2 The integration of carbohydrate and fat oxidation by skeletal muscle

The mechanisms by which muscle integrates the use of CHO and fat during prolonged exercise are complex and still unresolved. However, by way of example, it can be calculated that if the élite marathon runner depended solely on CHO as an energy source he would be exhausted after about 90 min of running. As the world record for the marathon is close to 130 min, this clearly exemplifies the importance of fuel integration during prolonged exercise.

It has been accepted for some time that the rate-limiting step in CHO oxidation is the decarboxylation of pyruvate to acetyl-CoA, which is controlled by the pyruvate dehydrogenase complex (PDH), and is essentially an irreversible reaction committing pyruvate to entry into the TCA cycle and oxidation. The PDH is a conglomerate of three enzymes located within the inner mitochondrial membrane. Adding to its complexity, the PDH also has two regulatory enzymes: a phosphatase and a kinase which regulate an activation/inactivation cycle. The phosphatase is responsible for dephosphorylating the PDH resulting in the transformation of the PDH to its active form (PDHa). Conversely, the kinase catalyses an ATP-dependent phosphorylation of the PDH with concomitant

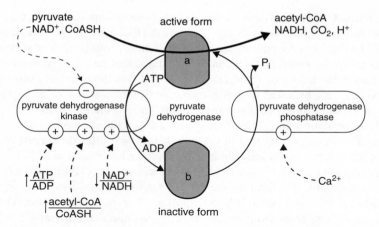

Fig. 7.1 The regulation of the pyruvate dehydrogenase complex. Activation (dephosphorylation) of pyruvate dehydrogenase by pyruvate dehydrogenase phosphatase and inactivation (phosphorylation) by pyruvate dehydrogenase kinase. Activation status is regulated via changes in calcium availability and alterations in the ATP:ADP, acetyl-CoA:CoA-SH, and NAD$^+$:NADH ratios.

inactivation of the enzyme complex. Interconversion of the PDH between its active to inactive form is regulated by several allosteric effectors and by hormonal action. Increased ratios of ATP/ADP, acetyl-CoA/CoA, and NADH/ NAD$^+$ activate the kinase, resulting in the inactivation of the enzyme. Conversely, decreases in the above ratios and the presence of pyruvate will inactivate the kinase, whilst increases in calcium will activate the phosphatase, together resulting in the activation of the PDH (Fig. 7.1) Thus, it can be seen that the increases in calcium and pyruvate availability at the onset of contraction will result in the rapid activation of the PDH. These factors, together with the subsequent decreases in the ATP/ADP, acetyl-CoA/CoA, and NADH/NAD$^+$ ratios as contraction continues, will result in continued flux through the reaction. Indeed, changes in these ratios can be seen to tightly regulate flux through the PDH reaction, such that pyruvate utilization will always parallel the demands of the TCA cycle and the electron transport chain. For example, assuming an adequate supply of ATP is achieved, a high mitochondrial ATP/ADP ratio would favour a reduction in the PDHa. Similarly, the inhibitory effect of an increased acetyl-CoA/CoA ratio on PDH activation ensures that the rate of acetyl-CoA formation does not outstrip the rate of acetyl group utilization by the TCA cycle. Finally, the inhibitory effect of an increased NADH/NAD$^+$ ratio will co-ordinate pyruvate oxidation with electron transport chain activity. This is, of course, an ideal scenario, which may not always be in operation. For example, recent evidence has shown that during maximal-intensity exercise with total blood flow occlusion, complete activation of the PDH occurs despite complete reduction of NAD$^+$ to NADH. This probably reflects two important points. First, that calcium availability and, therefore, exercise intensity is probably the most important regulator of PDH activation. Second, despite having complete activation of the enzyme, a very low flux rate through the PDH reaction can still occur.

With respect to acetyl-CoA accumulation during exercise, recent evidence indicates that an important role for carnitine (in addition to its role in the transport of long-chain fatty acids into the mitochondrial matrix) is in the buffering of excess acetyl group formation during exercise. In other words, when the rate of acetyl-CoA formation exceeds the rate at which the TCA cycle can re-cycle CoASH, free carnitine provides a sink for excess acetyl group formation (Fig. 7.2). For example, at exercise intensities below 30% $\dot{V}O_2$max acetylcarnitine formation is not usually observed, suggesting that the rate of acetyl-CoA formation is well matched by its rate of entry into the TCA cycle. However, as exercise intensity increases, acetylcarnitine accumulation has been found to occur in parallel with exercise intensity which is matched by a stoichiometric decline in free carnitine. This important role attributed to carnitine prevents the inhibition of many cellular processes which depend on a viable CoA pool, e.g. the PDH reaction and the TCA cycle at the level of α-ketoglutarate dehydrogenase.

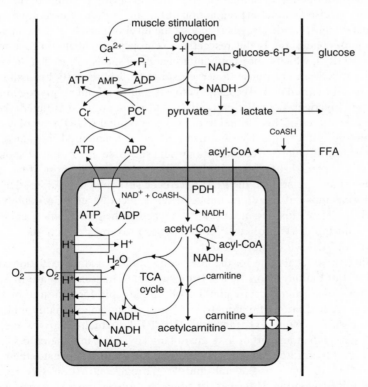

Fig. 7.2 The role of carnitine in buffering acetyl-group accumulation during intense contraction.

When considering the integration of CHO and fat oxidation by skeletal muscle, it is widely accepted that the accumulation of acetyl-CoA and NADH resulting from fat oxidation can reduce the amount of PDHa and its catalytic activity, thereby resulting in an inhibition of CHO oxidation. This interaction forms the basis of the glucose–fatty acid cycle proposed by Randle *et al.* (1963) which has, for many years, been accepted to be the key regulatory cycle in the integration of CHO and fat utilization by skeletal muscle. However, a growing body of evidence is accumulating to suggest that the glucose–fatty acid cycle does not operate in contracting human skeletal muscle. For example, recent work has demonstrated that when acetyl group availability has been forcibly increased using both intralipid and acetate infusion, consistent with the glucose–fatty acid cycle the PDHa was reduced at rest. However, during subsequent intense cycling exercise the decrease in the PDHa seen at rest following infusion was overcome, such that no differences in the PDHa were observed between the control and treatment groups. Despite this lack of an effect on the PDHa, muscle glycogen utilization during exercise was reduced by about 40% following intralipid infusion. This led to the proposal that the glucose–fatty acid cycle does not operate in human skeletal muscle during prolonged, moderate-intensity exercise and that the regulation of the integration of carbohydrate and fat oxidation must reside elsewhere, e.g. at the level of muscle glucose uptake or glycogen phosphorylase. In this respect, the neuropeptide calcitonin gene-related peptide (CGRP), which is present in motoneurones and is released at the neuro-muscular junction in response to nerve excitation, has recently been shown to inhibit insulin-stimulated glycogen synthesis and to stimulate glycogen phosphorylase, glycogen degradation, and lactate production in isolated skeletal muscle preparations. This has led to the suggestion that CGRP may play a role in regulating intracellular CHO utilization and is a potential mechanism for linking neuromuscular activation with muscle substrate utilization. It should be stressed, however, that the exercise intensities performed in most, if not all, of the above studies relating to the PDH have been sufficient to saturate PDH activation by calcium and, therefore, outweigh any effect of acetyl-CoA and NADH on PDH transformation. It is not yet known whether the glucose–fatty acid cycle operates during very prolonged, low-intensity exercise when the calcium activation of PDH will be at its lowest.

An alternative focal point for the integration of CHO and fat oxidation resides at the level of malonyl-CoA. It has been suggested that an increase in acetyl-CoA formation during exercise could result in the rapid formation of malonyl-CoA. The accumulation of malonyl-CoA has been shown to directly inhibit the enzyme carnitine palmitoyl transferase I (CPT I), which catalyses the rate-limiting step in the transport of long-chain fatty acyl-CoA into the mitochondria, which would therefore presumably decrease fat oxidation. To date, the role of malonyl-CoA in human skeletal muscle during contraction has received relatively little attention. However, its concentration has been shown to decline in rat skeletal muscle during contraction. The relevance of this finding to fuel substrate utilization is difficult to interpret because of a lack of other relevant data. Furthermore, because the sensitivity of rat muscle CPT I for malonyl-CoA is relatively high, it has been calculated that even at low malonyl-CoA concentrations, CPT I and, therefore, fat oxidation would be completely inhibited, which is clearly not the case. Undoubtedly, future research will provide us with more information as to the role of malonyl-CoA in the integration of fuel substrate utilization in exercising man.

7.3 Muscle carbohydrate availability, diet, and exercise

The CHO content of human skeletal muscle is about 350 mmol kg dm^{-1} and is fairly resistant to change in sedentary individuals. For example, increasing dietary CHO intake from about 55% of energy intake to 80–90% of energy intake will only increase muscle glycogen content by about 50 mmol kg dm^{-1}. Evidence suggests that this is due to the downregulation of the membrane glucose-transporter protein and glycogen synthase during conditions of adequate CHO supply. Similarly, 3–4 days of starvation will have little effect on the muscle glycogen store. This is unlike the response observed in other mammalian species. For example, the relatively high basal metabolic rate of the laboratory rat is too high to be met by fat oxidation alone and, therefore, 24 h of starvation will reduce the glycogen content of rat skeletal muscle to almost zero. Clearly, in the case of CHO metabolism, care should be taken when extrapolating results from animal studies to man.

The concept that CHO availability will limit exercise capacity during prolonged exercise has been a view accepted for most of this century. The pioneering work of Christensen and Hansen in the 1930s was the first to show that a CHO-rich diet during the days prior to prolonged exercise could increase exercise performance by 2–3 times compared with a fat-rich diet. Following the reintroduction of the use of the muscle-biopsy technique in the 1960s, Bergstrom and Hultman went on to demonstrate that a clear relationship exists between the pre-exercise muscle glycogen concentration and exercise performance. This work showed that a progressive decline in muscle glycogen concentration occurred during bicycle exercise at about 80% $\dot{V}O_2$max. After approximately 70 min of exercise the work rate could no longer be sustained and this coincided with muscle glycogen depletion (Fig. 7.3). At around this time, the same authors demonstrated that a combination of glycogen depletion and high dietary CHO intake could have a dramatic effect on muscle glycogen storage. It was demonstrated that following glycogen-depleting exercise, muscle glycogen stores could be increased to supranormal levels (about 900 mmol kg dm^{-1}) by ingesting a high CHO diet in the days following exercise (Fig. 7.4). The authors demonstrated that resynthesis was most rapid in the hours immediately following exercise, which was probably due to the activation of muscle glycogen synthase, the regulation of which has yet to be completely resolved. It was also clearly

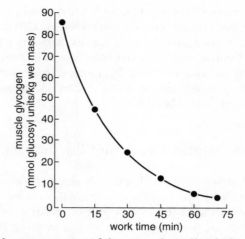

Fig. 7.3 Muscle glycogen content of the vastus lateralis of 10 subjects during bicycle exercise at an intensity equivalent to 80% V̇O₂max. On all occasions exercise was performed until voluntary exhaustion which coincided with the point of glycogen depletion. (From Bergstrom and Hultman, 1967a.)

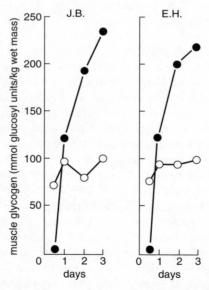

Fig. 7.4 Muscle glycogen content of the vastus lateralis muscle from previously inactive (○) and previously active (●) muscle of two subjects. Needle-biopsy samples were obtained immediately after one-legged bicycle exercise and for the following three days during which a high-carbohydrate diet was consumed. (From Bergstrom and Hultman, 1966.)

demonstrated that the supracompensation of muscle glycogen stores was restricted to the exercised muscle group. Further studies by the same authors showed a clear relationship between pre-exercise dietary intake, muscle glycogen stores, and exercise capacity. Muscle glycogen content was first altered by feeding different isoenergetic diets following glycogen-depleting exercise, after which the subjects cycled to the point of volitional exhaustion at a work rate equivalent to 75% $\dot{V}O_2$max. A normal mixed diet was given for the days prior to the first endurance test, a CHO-restricted diet before the second test, and a CHO-rich diet before the final test. Average muscle glycogen concentration following the normal-mixed, the CHO-restricted, and the CHO-rich diets were 495, 176, and 953 mmol kg dm^{-1} respectively. Looked at in another way, the CHO-restricted diet reduced muscle glycogen by about 65% and the CHO-rich diet increased it by about 95%. In parallel with these changes, exercise time to exhaustion was also changed. A close relationship was found between the pre-exercise muscle glycogen concentration and exercise time to exhaustion, and exhaustion always coincided with muscle glycogen depletion regardless of the preceding dietary regimen (Fig. 7.5). Thus, following the CHO-restricted diet the endurance time was reduced by about 55% to 59 min and following the CHO-rich diet increased by 50% to 180 min. One might have expected exercise time to have increased by more than 50% given the doubling of the muscle

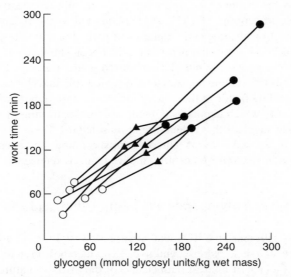

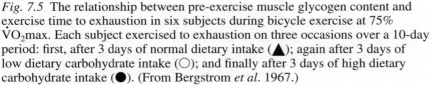

Fig. 7.5 The relationship between pre-exercise muscle glycogen content and exercise time to exhaustion in six subjects during bicycle exercise at 75% $\dot{V}O_2$max. Each subject exercised to exhaustion on three occasions over a 10-day period: first, after 3 days of normal dietary intake (▲); again after 3 days of low dietary carbohydrate intake (○); and finally after 3 days of high dietary carbohydrate intake (●). (From Bergstrom *et al.* 1967.)

glycogen store by prior to exercise. However, this reflects the common observation that muscle glycogen utilization is usually accelerated when muscle stores are elevated by exercise and dietary manipulation. This series of studies collectively represents one of the most significant research contributions to exercise science. In the 30 years that have passed since publication, these findings have been confirmed on many occasions, and the practice of 'carbohydrate loading' is now common amongst athletes world-wide. Indeed, a considerable amount of research funding has been devoted to optimizing the quantity and type of CHO to be ingested following exercise in an effort to maximize muscle glycogen resynthesis. However, the central message based on the work undertaken in the 1960s has not changed greatly, and research in the intervening years has principally been aimed at refining our understanding of the interaction between exercise, muscle glucose uptake, and metabolism. For example, it is now known that when a high-CHO diet is ingested during recovery from glycogen-depleting exercise, the rate of muscle glycogen resynthesis is about 25% greater in type I muscle fibres during the initial few hours of recovery. Following this, the rate of resynthesis appears to decline in Type I fibres, but is maintained in Type II fibres, such that 24 h following exercise there is no difference in the glycogen content between fibre types. The difference in glycogen resynthesis between fibre types during the initial part of recovery has been attributed to fibre type differences in the rates of membrane glucose transport which has been shown to be rate limited by the extent of incorporation of the insulin-responsive membrane-bound glucose transporter (GLUT 4). This has led to the recent proposal of insulin-dependent and-independent phases of glycogen resynthesis. The incorporation of GLUT 4 in muscle membranes has been shown to be increased by exercise and to be greatest in muscles composed predominantly of Type I fibres. Thus, this membrane protein appears to play a vital role in CHO metabolism and is likely to be a key factor in the widely reported improvement of whole-body insulin sensitivity which occurs as a result of exercise training. In this respect, recent evidence suggests that a decrease in muscle GLUT 4 content is responsible for the decreased rate of glucose transport and glycogen resynthesis observed following exercise-(eccentric) induced muscle damage.

7.4 Liver carbohydrate availability, diet, and exercise

In comparison with muscle CHO metabolism relatively little is known about the interaction between diet, exercise, and liver CHO metabolism in humans. This is not because of a lack of interest but because of the invasive nature of the liver-biopsy technique. The few studies that have been performed in healthy volunteers using this technique have demonstrated that the rate of liver glucose release in the postabsorptive state is in the region of 0.8–1.1 mmol of glucose min^{-1}, which is sufficient to meet the CHO demands of only the brain. Approximately 70% of this release (0.5 mmol min^{-1}) is derived from liver glycogen stores and the remainder is synthesized by gluconeogensis in the liver using lactate, pyruvate, glycerol, and amino acids as substrates. In the case of amino acids, it is appropriate to mention here the glucose–alanine cycle (Chapter 5). Experiments performed in the 1970s demonstrated that alanine was not just an end-product of muscle glycolysis (it is formed from the transamination of pyruvate), but it also contributed significantly to liver gluconeogenesis and served to maintain liver glucose production during conditions of CHO restriction. This led to the proposition of the existence of the glucose–alanine cycle operating between muscle and liver. The cycle involves alanine being synthesized from pyruvate and released by muscle. Circulating alanine is then extracted by the liver and its carbon skeleton is converted to glucose. Similarly, peripheral formation and hepatic extraction of glutamine has been demonstrated to operate in man, but this pathway seems to be less prevalent than that of alanine.

Liver-biopsy studies in man have clearly demonstrated that the liver is extremely sensitive to changes in dietary CHO intake. Based on the above measurements of the rates of glucose release in the postabsorptive state, it can be calculated that 1 day of starvation would completely empty the liver glycogen store. This was demonstrated by Nilsson and Hultman (1973) who showed that 1 day of starvation or CHO restriction depleted liver glycogen stores from about 270 to about 30 mmol kg wet mass^{-1}. Further CHO restriction maintained liver glycogen stores at this low level and approximately 50% of liver glucose released in this state was derived from gluconeogenesis. More recently, magnetic resonance spectroscopy studies have shown that liver gluconeogenesis accounts for about 65% of total-body glucose production during 22 h of fasting. Conversely, 1 day of high-dietary CHO intake can double the liver glycogen store to about 500 mmol kg wet mass of liver $^{-1}$ and less than 10% of the glucose released in this condition is derived from gluconeogenesis.

The rate of hepatic glucose release during exercise in the postabsorptive state has been shown to be mainly a function of exercise intensity. However, following a high-CHO diet the rate of release has been shown to increase. The uptake of gluconeogenic precursors by the liver increases 2–3 fold during exercise but most (approximately 90%) of the glucose released is derived from liver glycogenolysis, resulting in a decline and ultimately depletion of liver glycogen stores. It is known that the decline in blood insulin concentration and increases in adrenaline and glucagon with increasing exercise duration will stimulate liver glucose release. However, the exact mechanisms responsible for the regulation of liver glucose release at the onset and during exercise are still unresolved. It would appear that glucose release begins almost immediately at the onset of exercise and is initiated by a mechanism(s) which is sensitive to both the onset and intensity of muscle contraction. One widely accepted theory implicates a decline in local blood glucose concentration at the onset of exercise with the activation of liver phosphorylase, either directly or via hormonal stimulation. However, most studies have demonstrated an increase in blood glucose concentration at the onset of exercise, thereby refuting this theory. Other suggested, but just as inconclusive, regulatory mechanisms include hormonal and autonomic stimulation. With the recent technological developments in whole-body magnetic resonance spectroscopy it is hoped that more conclusive information concerning the regulation of liver CHO metabolism will soon become available. What is clear, however, is that during exercise at about 60% $\dot{V}O_2max$ glucose output from the liver will begin to decline after about 90 min of exercise as the liver glycogen stores become depleted. It has also been shown that the rate of liver glycogen resynthesis is dependent on the form of CHO presented to the liver. For example, resynthesis is 3–4 times faster when fructose is infused compared with glucose. This is because of the very high activity of fructokinase in liver tissue. This has important implications for exercise performance as the liver is the only significant source of blood glucose. Studies using animals and human volunteers have shown that liver glycogen depletion during exercise can limit performance either indirectly, by bringing about a more rapid depletion of muscle glycogen stores, or directly, by bringing about the development of hypoglycaemia which will inhibit neurological function. With this in mind, it is appropriate to maximize both muscle and liver CHO stores prior to prolonged exercise.

7.5 Carbohydrate ingestion immediately prior to exercise

The ingestion of CHO prior to exercise will help ensure that liver glycogen stores are 'optimal'. However, work in the 1970s, suggesting that CHO ingested prior to exercise was detrimental to exercise performance, resulted in pre-exercise CHO intake being avoided by athletes for many years. This effect was attributed to a transient increase in blood glucose levels following CHO ingestion thus bringing about a rapid release of insulin, and resulting in a decline in blood glucose concentration, the inhibition of free fatty-acid release, and the early development of fatigue (the insulin-rebound effect). With hindsight, it is clearer today that this response may have been mediated by the large amounts of CHO ingested prior to exercise (about 75 g, 30–45 min before exercise). More recent studies have shown that the ingestion of smaller amounts of CHO just before exercise result in no elevation of plasma insulin during exercise, no rebound hypoglycaemia, and an improvement in performance. As a result of this, the ingestion of CHO solutions prior to exercise has become more common.

As stated earlier, fructose has been suggested as a source of CHO to be ingested immediately prior to exercise. This is apparently because, compared with glucose, it results in little insulin release, a lower rate of muscle glycogen utilization, and a 3–4 fold acceleration of liver glycogen synthesis. However, studies to date, investigating the effect of fructose ingestion on muscle glycogen utilization and performance, have been equivocal, which may be attributable to the gastrointestinal discomfort reported to occur following fructose ingestion. This highlights an important point: it is not advisable to take findings from highly controlled laboratory studies and apply them directly to the athletic arena. Such practices should be tried and tested in training before being practised in competition as there may be a considerable interindividual variation in the tolerance to CHO drinks.

7.6 Carbohydrate ingestion during exercise

It has been known since the 1930s that the ingestion of CHO during exercise can increase endurance capacity during prolonged exercise. More recently, this has been attributed to CHO ingestion preserving muscle glycogen stores. This was clearly demonstrated in an experiment performed by Bergstrom and Hultman (1967b) which is often overlooked today. The authors demonstrated that the intravenous infusion of glucose into untrained subjects over the course of 70 min exercise at 70% of $\dot{V}O_2$max could reduce muscle glycogen utilization by 25%. One important point, however, is that the glucose infusion in this study resulted in an increase in blood glucose concentration from 4.6 to 21.5 mmol litre^{-1}, which is somewhat non-physiological. More recent studies have demonstrated that an increase in blood glucose by 2–3 mmol litre^{-1} during exercise as a result of CHO ingestion can increase exercise performance. In the vast majority of cases, CHO ingestion during exercise has been found to increase CHO oxidation during exercise; as might be expected, fat mobilization and oxidation is decreased. It seems clear, therefore, that for CHO ingestion during exercise to be successful in reducing muscle glycogen utilization and improving exercise performance, its contribution to total energy production must be greater than that derived from fat oxidation. More recent work has demonstrated that the glycogen sparing effect of CHO ingestion during prolonged exercise appears to be restricted solely to Type I muscle fibres. Tsintzas *et al.* (1996) demonstrated that, compared with placebo ingestion, CHO ingestion was associated with a 25% reduction of glycogen utilization in Type I muscle fibres following 104 min of exercise. Glycogen utilization in Type II fibres was unaffected by CHO ingestion. Furthermore, the ingestion of CHO enabled a further 30 min of exercise to be performed. The authors concluded that CHO ingestion improved endurance capacity by contributing to oxidative ATP production specifically in Type I muscle fibres and by so doing delayed the development of glycogen depletion in this fibre type.

It is also important to remember that even if muscle glycogen utilization is unaffected by CHO ingestion, it may still favourably affect exercise performance by postponing the rate of liver glycogen depletion, or taking the place of liver glycogen stores when they become depleted, thereby delaying the onset of hypoglycaemia. Indeed, an increase in exercise time to exhaustion has been associated with the improved maintenance of blood glucose levels on several occasions. In one classic study performed by Coyle *et al.* (1986) the authors demonstrated that there was no difference in muscle glycogen utilization during

3 h of exercise when subjects were fed a flavoured placebo or a glucose polymer solution every 20 min during exercise. However, when the subjects ingested the placebo solution they became exhausted after 182 min, blood glucose concentration fell to 2.5 mmol litre^{-1} towards the end of exercise, and this was accompanied by a decline in CHO oxidation. In contrast, when the glucose solution was ingested, the subjects exercised for over 240 min and euglycaemia and CHO oxidation were maintained throughout. Furthermore, the additional hour of exercise was performed with little utilization of muscle glycogen stores. Presumably this was because the activity of hexokinase (the enzyme responsible for phosphorylating glucose at the muscle membrane) was increased. This response probably occurred because the inhibitory effect of hexosemonophosphates on hexokinase activity declined as the muscle glycogen store became increasingly depleted. The authors concluded from this study that the ingestion of CHO during exercise increases endurance time principally by maintaining CHO oxidation from blood glucose rather than by sparing muscle glycogen stores. One word of caution, however. This study was performed using highly trained endurance athletes and it is unclear whether such high rates of glucose oxidation could be maintained from circulatory sources in untrained individuals.

7.7 The effect of increasing fat availability prior to exercise

Fat oxidation has the ability to provide all the muscle energy requirements during highly prolonged, low-intensity exercise (less than 40% maximal oxygen consumption). However, in order to avoid hypoglycaemia during this type of exercise, hepatic glucose production must be maintained. For these reasons, dietary intake has been of interest to military personnel involved in long-term activity. In one particular study, subjects walked for about 40 km day^{-1} for 4 days; during this time CHO constituted about 3% of their total energy intake. Although the utilization of fat was increased during this period, at no point did any of the subjects become hypoglycaemic and all subjects completed the exercise task (Fig. 7.6). It would appear that, similar to resting conditions, liver glycogenolysis and gluconeogenesis can match the CHO demands of this type of exercise.

On a weight to weight basis, lipid is approximately 5-fold more efficient than CHO as a storage fuel and the body store of lipid can be considered as inexhaustible, and therefore, in terms of energy supply there would be distinct advantages if fat was the principal fuel oxidized during prolonged exercise. In this respect, the improvement in exercise capacity seen after endurance training has been attributed by some to an increased contribution from fat oxidation reducing the rate of glycogen depletion. This has led to the hypothesis that a fat-loading dietary regimen prior to exercise can improve exercise performance. Presumably, this mechanism would work by inhibiting the catalytic activity of the PDH, and thereby reducing CHO oxidation during exercise (the glucose–

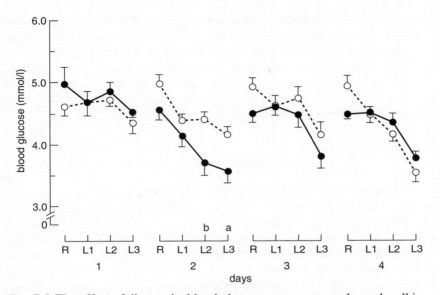

Fig. 7.6 The effect of diet on the blood glucose response to prolonged walking on consecutive days. Mean ± SE values of blood glucose concentration before and during high-CHO (open circles) and low-CHO (closed circles) diets. R refers to the fasting pre-exercise sample each day and L1, L2, and L3 refer to samples obtained after completion of laps 1, 2 and 3, respectively. Each lap was approximately 13 km in distance and was covered at a constant speed (From Maughan *et al.* 1987.)

fatty acid cycle). However, as stated previously, there is very little evidence to suggest that the glucose–fatty acid cycle operates in human skeletal muscle during intense exercise. Furthermore, while this strategy may be effective for the rat, there is very little data to support the concept of fat loading in man. Instead, the literature currently suggests that physical and psychological performance are more likely to be impaired by attempting to increase fat availability. Indeed, as stated earlier, and based on empirical measurements, it is clear that fat oxidation alone could not sustain ATP at the rate required to maintain energy delivery during prolonged exercise in man at a work rate greater than about 60% $\dot{V}O_2$max.

In a number of studies, caffeine ingestion (3–9 mg kg body mass^{-1}) prior to exercise has been reported to increase endurance capacity during prolonged cycling exercise. The increase in free fatty-acid mobilization as a result of caffeine ingestion, together with the subsequent reduction in muscle glycogen utilization during exercise, has led to the suggestion that caffeine's ergogenic effect is attributable to the increase in fat availability. However, this mechanism of action has not been demonstrated to occur. Indeed, no mechanism has yet been clearly established. Alternative candidates include a direct effect of caffeine on the central nervous system and/or on the excitation/contraction coupling mechanism. In the case of the latter, caffeine has been shown to stimulate the re-uptake of calcium by the sarcoplasmic reticulum *in vitro*.

7.8 Fatigue mechanisms

Despite the wealth of information showing that CHO availability is essential to performance during intense prolonged exercise, the exact biochemical mechanism(s) by which fatigue is brought about in the CHO-depleted state are still unclear. Recent evidence suggests that CHO depletion will result in an inability to rephosphorylate ADP to ATP at the required rate, and that the consequent rise in ADP concentration will bring about fatigue, perhaps as a direct inhibitory effect of ADP and/or P_i on excitation-contraction coupling. Support for this hypothesis comes from two different experimental lines of evidence. First, it has been demonstrated that when CHO stores become depleted, the concentration of muscle TCA-cycle intermediates declines, and, as a consequence, it has been suggested that this may decrease the rate of flux through the TCA cycle and thereby decrease oxidative ATP resynthesis. The administration of glucose during exercise has been shown to diminish the decline in the concentration of TCA-cycle intermediates towards the end of exercise, thereby maintaining the muscle ATP:ADP ratio and delaying fatigue development. Presumably, the administration of CHO ensures that the availability of pyruvate does not limit the rate of flux through the anaplerotic reaction responsible for the generation of the TCA-cycle intermediate 2-oxoglutarate (pyruvate + glutamate → 2-oxoglutarate + alanine). The second line of evidence, suggesting that CHO depletion will bring about fatigue due to an increase in ADP, comes from studies showing that in muscle in the glycogen-depleted state the ATP concentration declines and is matched by a stoichiometric increase in the concentrations of ADP and IMP. Muscle fatigue and the increase in IMP concentration occur because of the inability of oxidative phosphorylation to rephosphorylate ADP to ATP, resulting in the activation of AMP deaminase and the formation of IMP.

Thus, it would appear that CHO availability is essential for the continuation of exercise, since fatigue development will occur when it becomes impossible to maintain the rate of rephosphorylation of ADP to ATP in the glycogen-depleted state. This is consistent with the hypothesis that fatigue is due to an increase in the intracellular ADP concentration inhibiting excitation–contraction coupling. It is also worth noting that the energy yield during ATP hydrolysis decreases when the products of its hydrolysis (ADP and P_i) increase in concentration which may also accelerate the development of fatigue by impairing ATP utilizing reactions.

This chapter has been concerned with the metabolic responses to prolonged exercise and, therefore, little attention has been given to fluid balance during exercise. However, it is perhaps worth noting at this point that dehydration could arguably be the most important factor in the development of fatigue during prolonged exercise in man, especially in a hot and humid environment. The rise in core temperature that occurs during prolonged exercise in a hot environment is potentially life-threatening and the increase in skin blood flow and the onset of sweating under these conditions is the body's attempt to increase heat loss. The maintenance of adequate hydration has been shown to attenuate the increase in core temperature during exercise. However, with the development of dehydration, increased stress is placed upon the cardiovascular and thermoregulatory systems to maintain heat balance. Furthermore, recent evidence suggests that a decrease in muscle blood flow under these conditions may accelerate the rate of muscle glycogen utilization which will presumably augment the early development of fatigue. Research has shown that dehydration is relatively common amongst athletes and impairs exercise performance by mechanisms yet to be completely resolved. It has also become clear that maintaining hydration during exercise can reduce the physiological stresses associated with dehydration and improve exercise performance. Consequently, the consumption of weak glucose–electrolyte solutions has become common amongst endurance athletes.

7.9 Key points

1. The term 'prolonged exercise' is usually used to describe exercise intensities that can be sustained for between 30 and 180 min. Since the rate of ATP demand is relatively low compared with high-intensity exercise, PCr, CHO, and fat can all contribute to energy production.

2. The rates of PCr degradation and lactate production during the first minutes of prolonged exercise are closely related to the intensity of exercise performed, and it is likely that energy production during this period would be compromised without this contribution from anaerobic metabolism. However, once a steady state has been reached, CHO and fat become the principal substrates.

3. Under normal conditions, muscle CHO stores alone could fuel about 80 min of exercise before becoming depleted. However, the simultaneous utilization of body fat and hepatic CHO stores enables ATP production to be maintained and exercise to continue. Ultimately, though, ATP production becomes compromised due to the muscle and hepatic CHO stores becoming depleted and the inability of fat oxidation to increase to offset this deficit. It is currently unknown which factor limits the maximal rate of fat oxidation during exercise (i.e why it cannot increase to compensate for CHO depletion), but it must precede acetyl-CoA formation as from this point fat and carbohydrate share the same fate.

4. It is generally accepted that the glucose–fatty acid cycle regulates the integration of CHO and fat oxidation during prolonged exercise. However, whilst this may be true of resting muscle, recent evidence suggests that the cycle does not operate in exercising muscle and that the site of regulation must reside elsewhere (e.g. at the level of phosphorylase and/or malonyl-CoA). From the literature it would appear that the integration of muscle CHO and fat utilization during prolonged exercise is complex and unresolved.

5. In sedentary individuals the CHO store of human muscle is fairly resistant to change. However, the combination of exercise and dietary manipulation can have dramatic effects on subsequent muscle CHO storage. Furthermore, a clear positive relationship has been shown to exist between muscle CHO content and subsequent prolonged exercise performance.

6. Starvation will rapidly deplete the liver of CHO, but has little effect on skeletal muscle. The rate of hepatic glucose release in resting postabsorptive individuals is sufficient to match the CHO demands of only the central nervous system. Approximately 70% of this release is derived from liver CHO stores and the remainder from liver gluconeogenesis. During exercise, the rate of hepatic glucose release has been shown to be related to exercise intensity. Of this release, 90% is derived from liver CHO stores, ultimately resulting in liver glycogen depletion. The exact mechanisms responsible for the regulation of hepatic glucose release during exercise are unresolved. Hepatic glucose uptake following exercise has been shown to be, at least partly, dependent on the form of CHO presented to the liver.

7. The ingestion of CHO during the hours before exercise will ensure that hepatic CHO stores are optimal. There is no reason to believe such procedures will impair exercise performance as a result of the insulin-rebound effect. Indeed, it is now generally accepted that CHO ingestion prior to prolonged exercise will improve performance.

8. The ingestion of CHO during prolonged exercise has been shown to decrease muscle glycogen utilization and fat mobilization and oxidation, and to increase CHO oxidation and endurance capacity during prolonged exercise. It is clear, therefore, that the contribution of ingested CHO to total energy production under these conditions must be greater than that normally derived from fat oxidation. Evidence suggests that CHO ingestion during prolonged exercise exerts its main functional and metabolic effects on Type I muscle fibres. Carbohydrate ingestion could also retard fatigue development by delaying the rate of liver glycogen depletion and, thereby, the development of hypoglycaemia during exercise.

9. The improvement in exercise capacity following endurance training has been interpreted by some to be due to an increase in fat oxidation reducing muscle glycogen utilization. This has led to the hypothesis that fat ingestion prior to exercise will improve endurance capacity. However, the maximal rate of fat oxidation is insufficient to match the rate of ATP resynthesis required during prolonged exercise at more than 60% $\dot{V}O_2$max and, as might be expected therefore, performance has usually been found to be impaired under these conditions.

10. The exact biochemical mechanism by which muscle CHO depletion results in fatigue is presently unresolved. However, it is plausible that the inability of muscle to maintain the rate of ADP rephosphorylation in the glycogen-depleted state results in ADP and P_i accumulation and, consequently, fatigue development.

Further reading

Broberg, S. and Sahlin, K. (1989). Adenine nucleotide degradation in human skeletal muscle during prolonged exercise. *J. Appl. Physiol.*, **67**, 116–22.

Coyle, E. F., Hadberg, J. M., Hurley, B. F., Martin, W. H., Ehsani, A. A., and Holloszy, J. O. (1983). Carbohydrate feeding during prolonged strenuous exercise can delay fatigue. *J. Appl. Physiol.*, **55**, 230–5.

Dyke, D. J., Putman, C. T., Heigenhauser, G. J. F., Hultman, E., and Spriet, L. L. (1993). Regulation of fat–carbohydrate interaction in skeletal muscle during intense aerobic cycling. *Am. J. Physiol.*, **265**, E852–E859.

Putman, C. T., Spriet, L. L., Hultman, E., Dyke, D. J., and Heigenhauser, G. J. F. (1995). Skeletal muscle pyruvate dehydrogenase activity during acetate infusion in humans. *Am. J. Physiol*, **268**, E1007–E1017.

Sahlin, K., Katz, A., and Broberg, S. (1990). Tricarboxylic cycle intermediates in human muscle during submaximal exercise. *Am. J. Physiol.*, **259**, C834–C841.

References

Bergstrom, J. and Hultman, E. (1966). Muscle glycogen synthesis after exercise: an enhancing factor localised to the muscle cells in man. *Nature*, **1210**, 309–10.

Bergstrom, J. and Hultman, E. (1967a). A study of glycogen metabolism during exercise in man. *Scand. J. Clin. Lab. Invest.*, **19**, 218–28.

Bergstrom, J. and Hultman, E. (1967b). Synthesis of muscle glycogen in man after glucose and fructose infusion. *Acta Med. Scand.*, **182**, 93–107.

Bergstrom, J., Hermansen, L., Hultman, E., and Saltin, B. (1967). Diet, muscle glycogen and physical performance. *Acta Physiol. Scand.*, **71**, 140–50.

Coyle, E. F., Coggan, A. R., Hemmert, M. K., and Ivy, J. L. (1986). Muscle glycogen utilisation during prolonged strenuous exercise when fed carbohydrate. *J. Appl. Physiol.*, **61**, 165–72.

Maughan, R. J., Greenhaff, P. L., Gleeson, M., Fenn, C. E., and Leiper, J. B. (1987). The effect of dietary carbohydrate intake on the metabolic response to prolonged walking on consecutive days. *Eur. J. Appl. Physiol.*, **56**, 583–91.

Nilsson, L. H. and Hultman, E. (1973). Liver glycogen in man—the effect of total starvation or a carbohydrate-poor diet followed by carbohydrate feedings. *Scand. J. Clin. Lab. Invest.*, **32**, 325–30.

Randle, P. J., Garland, P. B., Hales, C. N., and Newsholme, E. A. (1963). The glucose fatty acid cycle: its role in insulin sensitivity and the metabolic disturbances of diabetes mellitus. *Lancet*, 786–9.

Tsintzas, O.-K., Williams, C., Boobis, L., and Greenhaff, P. L. (1996). Carbohydrate ingestion and single muscle fibre glycogen metabolism during prolonged running in man. *J. Appl. Physiol.*, **81**, 801–9.

8
Metabolic adaptation to training

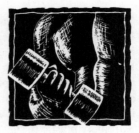

8.1 Principles of training

Both physiological and biochemical adaptations occur as a result of performing repeated bouts of exercise over several days, weeks, or months. These adaptations improve performance in specific tasks. The nature and magnitude of the adaptive response is dependent on the intensity and duration of exercise bouts, the mode of training and the frequency of repetition of the activity, genetic limitations, and the level of prior activity of the individual.

In order to bring about effective adaptation a specific and repeated exercise overload must be applied. A general principle (Table 8.1) is that adaptation to training will only occur if the person exercises at a level above their normal habitual level of activity on a frequent basis. The appropriate overload for any individual can be achieved by manipulating combinations of training intensity, duration, frequency, and mode. Another important principle is that physiological and metabolic adaptations to training are generally specific to the nature of the exercise overload. Training for speed and strength induces adaptations that are different from those elicited by endurance training. The major effects of endurance training on skeletal muscle are on its oxidative capacity and its capillary supply. Strength training, on the other hand, mainly influences the size (cross-sectional area) of a muscle and thus its force-generating capacity. The specific exercise mode is also important: for example, the development of endurance capacity for running, cycling, swimming, or rowing is most effectively achieved when training involves the specific muscles used in the desired activity. This is because regular exercise induces adaptations that are both central (e.g. improvements in cardiac performance) and peripheral (e.g. improvements in local muscular performance).

Table 8.1   Principles of training

Overload:	Frequency, mode, intensity, and duration of exercise
Specificity:	Muscles engaged in activity endurance or strength training
Individual response:	Initial fitness
	Genetic limitations
Reversible and transient effects	
Overtraining:	Time for regenerative recovery required

Adaptations to training are essentially transient and reversible: after only a few days of detraining, significant reductions in both metabolic and work capacity are demonstrable and many of the training improvements are lost within a few months of stopping regular exercise. Excessive training loads may cause breakdown and loss of performance, a condition referred to as the 'overtraining syndrome'. Sufficient time for regenerative recovery is required within a training programme to allow morphological adaptations to occur. Muscle is an extremely plastic tissue, and although genetic factors are the major determinant of the quantity and quality of muscle present in an untrained individual, considerable changes in the functional characteristics, morphology, and metabolic capacity can be induced by training.

The reader is referred to some excellent texts that review the central adaptations to endurance training. In this chapter the emphasis will be placed on local adaptations occurring in skeletal muscle in response to endurance or speed/power/strength type training.

8.2 Adaptation to endurance training

Endurance overload training involving exercise at 50–80% $\dot{V}O_2$max for prolonged periods, performed several times per week, induces adaptations that significantly improve functional capacities related to oxygen delivery, uptake, and use. These adaptations are summarized in Table 8.2.

The ability to maintain prolonged dynamic exercise such as cycling or running is dependent on the rate of ATP utilization within the active muscle being matched by the rate of ATP supply; if this is not the case, then fatigue ensues: the rate of ATP use must fall and hence the power output declines. During any exercise which can be sustained for more than a few minutes, the majority of the ATP provision is supplied by oxidative phosphorylation in the mitochondria, involving the utilization of carbohydrate and lipid fuels. This process requires an adequate supply of oxygen, delivered by the blood, and adequate fuel. The latter may be derived from within the muscle fibre (glycogen

---

Table 8.2   Muscle adaptation to endurance training

Selective hypertrophy of Type I fibres
Increased number of blood capillaries per muscle fibre
Increased myoglobin content
Increased capacity of mitochondria to generate ATP by oxidative phosphorylation
Increased size and number of mitochondria
Increased capacity to oxidize lipid and carbohydrate
Increased reliance on lipid as fuel
Higher glycogen and triglyceride content
Increased endurance capacity

---

and triglyceride) or from the circulation (glucose and FFA). Disruption of the ATP supply can arise if the intramuscular fuel depots become exhausted or if the circulation fails to provide sufficient fuels or oxygen. The regular performance of endurance exercise causes muscular and cardiovascular adaptations that influence these processes and thus determine fuel and oxygen provision. These adaptations, which include ultrastructural as well as metabolic (enzymatic) changes, lead to an improved capacity for oxygen delivery to and its extraction by the active musculature, as well as a modified and improved control of metabolism within the individual muscle fibres. A discussion of these changes that occur in response to endurance training follows.

8.2.1 Fibre type composition

Fibre type composition is clearly different in élite endurance-trained and strength-trained athletes. Type I fibres predominate in successful endurance athletes, whereas top-class sprinters have muscles containing mostly Type II fibres. Costill *et al.* (1976) found that 79% of the muscle fibres in the gastrocnemius muscle of élite distance runners could be classified as Type I fibres, with a range from 50 to 98%; non-élite middle-distance runners had a mean of 62% Type I fibres and untrained men a mean of 58% Type I fibres. Not only were the élite runners' Type I fibres more numerous than the Type II fibres, they were also 30% larger in terms of their individual fibre cross-sectional area; this meant that 83% of the total muscle cross-sectional area was occupied by Type I fibres. Type I and Type II fibres were the same size in the other two groups of subjects. Longitudinal studies have confirmed that endurance training can influence the size of individual muscle fibres, causing a selective hypertrophy of Type I fibres, and can also dramatically enhance their oxidative capacity. Training can have a strong influence on the functional and metabolic properties of muscle and its component fibres, and there is strong evidence from studies in animals and man that fibre type transformations can occur in response to cross-innervation or prolonged electrical stimulation. Both intense endurance and interval training have also been reported to alter muscle fibre composition in the rat. There is some evidence that relatively modest training programmes can induce a measurable alteration in fibre composition in man (Table 8.3). Andersen and Henriksson (1977) reported that 8 weeks of endurance training resulted in the conversion of some Type IIb fibres to Type IIa: this would be consistent with reports that endurance athletes have only a few Type IIb fibres. However, these changes in muscle fibre composition in response to endurance training seem quite small. In general, it seems that at least part of the success of endurance athletes (e.g. marathon runners), including the high proportion of Type I fibres found in their muscles (typically 70–90%), can be attributed to favourable genetic endowment, rather than an adaptation to training.

Table 8.3   Training-induced changes in muscle fibre composition

Fibre type	Before[a]	After[a]	Before[b]	After[b]
I	41	43	58	57
IIa	37	42*	26	32*
IIb	19	14*	9	3*

* Significantly different from before training ($p < 0.005$)
[a] Data from Andersen and Henriksson (1977)
[b] Data from Ingjer (1979)

Many of the studies that have reported changes in muscle fibre composition in response to training have taken no account of possible differential changes in the sizes of the different muscle fibre types following training. Simoneau *et al.* (1985), however, found that 15 weeks of high-intensity interval training resulted in an increase in the proportion of Type I fibres and a decrease in the proportion of Type II fibres, with no change in the number of Type IIa fibres; the cross-sectional area of fibres classified as Types I and IIb increased. Changes in the proportions of the different fibre types present after training cannot, therefore, be accounted for by changes in fibre area alone.

There is obviously a limit to the extent that muscle fibres can grow in diameter. This may be partly because with increasing diameter the distance that oxygen must diffuse is also increased. Improvements in capillary density could partly offset this limitation, however, allowing some degree of fibre hypertrophy without markedly affecting the average oxygen diffusion distance.

8.2.2 Muscle capillary density

Both cross-sectional (Fig. 8.1) and longitudinal studies (Fig. 8.2) indicate that endurance training increases the capillary density of skeletal muscle, expressed as the number of capillaries per fibre and as the number of capillaries per unit area. The capillary bed of muscle plays a crucial role in providing a surface for exchange between muscle and blood. Increasing the number of capillaries surrounding individual muscle fibres will mean that when a fibre is recruited it becomes more effectively exposed to the flow of blood delivered to the muscle during exercise. Thus, improvements in capillary density potentially allow an improved rate of transfer of oxygen, nutrients, and waste products at high perfusion rates by presenting a greater surface area for diffusion and by shortening the average diffusion distance. More than 99% of the oxygen in blood is transported by the haemoglobin in the red blood cells. Increased capillarity would also be expected to slow down the blood flow rate through the capillaries at any given rate of total tissue blood flow, and this could increase the length of time available for the diffusion of oxygen to occur (i.e. each red blood cell spends more time in the capillary). This effect may be crucial since it appears that

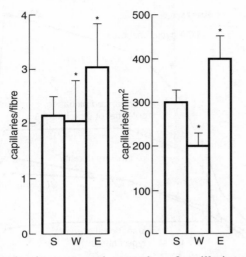

Fig. 8.1 Capillary density expressed as number of capillaries per muscle fibre and number of capillaries per unit area (mm²) of vastus lateralis muscle in sedentary controls (S), weightlifters (W), and endurance athletes (E). * Significantly different from sedentary subjects ($p < 0.01$). Values are means ± SD. (From Tesch *et al.* 1984.)

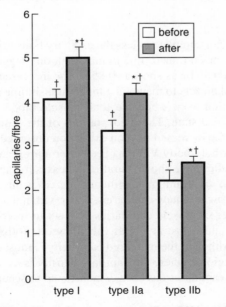

Fig. 8.2 Changes in capillary density surrounding different fibre types in vastus lateralis muscle before and after endurance training. * Significantly different than before training ($p < 0.01$). † Significantly different from other fibre types in the same condition ($p < 0.01$). Values are means ± SEM. (From Ingjer 1979.)

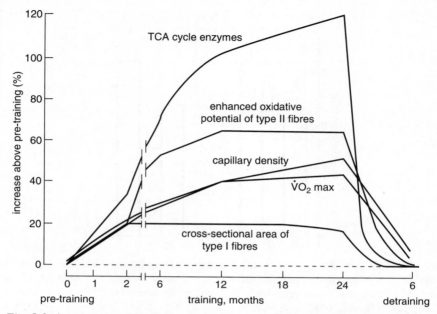

Fig. 8.3 A summary of the time course of some of the adaptations taking place in skeletal muscle during endurance training and subsequent inactivity (detraining).

oxygen extraction is not complete unless the capillary transit time is close to one second, whereas the mean transit time in maximal, one-legged exercise is less than half of this and may be as short as 0.25 s. The increased capillary density will allow the trained muscle to maintain a longer transit time and thus achieve a high oxygen extraction even when the total muscle blood flow is increased relative to the untrained state. These adaptations of the vasculature could, no doubt, contribute to the increased oxygen extraction observed in trained muscle and the increase in whole-body $\dot{V}O_2$max seen after a programme of endurance training. Several studies have shown parallel increases in capillary density and $\dot{V}O_2$max in response to training; significant increases in capillary density, resulting from the growth of new capillaries, occur within the first few weeks of training. The number of muscle capillaries appears to increase progressively throughout training and is lost at a relatively slow rate following cessation of training (Fig. 8.3). Although the increased capillarity is most easily observed in the Type IIb fibre regions, where the capillary density is usually the least, this development of new capillaries has been demonstrated to occur in all fibre types.

8.2.3 Muscle myoglobin content

Animal studies have indicated that the skeletal muscle content of myoglobin may increase by up to about 80% after training. Hence, the potential of the resting muscle fibre to store oxygen is increased. However, this is considered to be of relatively minor importance in contributing to the improvement of oxidative capacity with training. The main effect of an increased myoglobin content is likely to occur during exercise and be associated with the maintenance of a low pO_2 in the sarcoplasm of the muscle fibre, facilitating the diffusion of oxygen into the muscle from the blood. However, there appears to be no increase in the myoglobin content of human skeletal muscle with training and there may even be a decrease.

8.2.4 Intramuscular fuel stores

Numerous studies have reported that well-trained individuals have a higher muscle glycogen content at rest (up to 2.5 times the muscle glycogen content compared with before training). This increase in glycogen storage may be due, in part, to the increased sensitivity to insulin induced by training. This promotes glucose uptake (GLUT 4 transporter protein levels are 25% higher in trained muscle) and storage; whole-body, non-oxidative glucose disposal during glucose infusion has been reported to be about 60% higher in endurance-trained athletes than in sedentary controls, with only the trained men showing a significant storage of glucose as glycogen in skeletal muscle. The activity of glycogen synthase (both total and insulin-stimulated) is higher after training, although the activity of enzymes concerned with glycogen breakdown (phosphorylase) is also increased. Treadmill training studies in rats indicate a 20–40% increase in muscle hexokinase activity after training. Insulin also stimulates increases in the blood flow to insulin-sensitive tissues in a dose-responsive manner, and, as trained muscle possesses improved capillarity, this effect of insulin could enhance glucose delivery to trained muscle. These findings suggest that trained muscle develops an enhanced capacity for glucose storage as glycogen. However, the muscle glycogen concentration will obviously depend on the time since the last training bout and the subsequent dietary intake of carbohydrate. Higher muscle glycogen contents in trained individuals may reflect the phenomenon of glycogen supercompensation. Several studies have also reported a considerably higher intramuscular triacylglycerol content in trained individuals compared with untrained controls. Hence, the availability of both carbohydrate and lipid substrate appears to be higher after training, provided that sufficient time has elapsed since the last exercise bout to allow intramuscular fuel stores to be replenished.

8.2.5 Glycolytic capacity

Relatively little information is available concerning the effects of endurance training on glycolytic capacity compared with aerobic capacity. Although a few human studies have indicated that some of the key enzymes of glycolysis, including phosphofructokinase, are increased by about 20% following training,

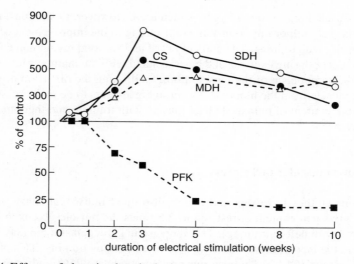

Fig. 8.4 Effects of chronic electrical stimulation on the activities of phosphofructokinase (PFK), the rate-limiting enzyme in the glycolytic pathway, and mitochondrial TCA cycle enzymes, citrate synthase (CS), malate dehydrogenase (MDH), succinate dehydrogenase (SDH). (From Henriksson *et al.* 1986.)

it must be said that most others have reported either no change or slight decreases in the activity of glycolytic enzymes after aerobic exercise training in both rats and humans. The content of glycolytic enzymes in the muscles of endurance athletes is usually found to be low, but this finding can be largely explained by their high percentage of Type I fibres which have a low glycolytic capacity compared with the Type II fibres. During chronic electrical stimulation of rabbit muscle, which induced a complete transformation of Type IIb to Type I fibres, the glycolytic enzyme content of the muscle decreased to only 20% of the initial level (Fig. 8.4), which reflects the rather large difference in glycolytic potential between fast-twitch and slow-twitch fibres in the rabbit. During periods of electrical stimulation, the oxidative enzyme capacity of muscle has been shown to increase to over 300% of the initial level. Such studies reveal the maximal capacity for biochemical adaptation in skeletal muscle.

8.2.6 Muscle mitochondrial density and oxidative enzyme activity

Mitochondria from trained muscle have a greatly increased capacity to generate ATP aerobically by oxidative phosphorylation. The oxidative capacity of skeletal muscle is also enhanced by a marked increase in both the size and number of mitochondria per unit area (Fig. 8.5) and an increase in the membrane surface

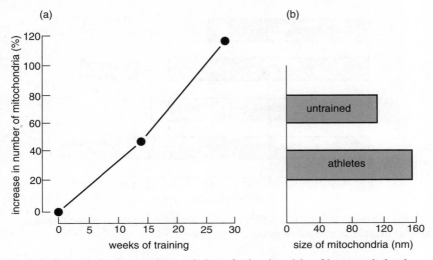

Fig. 8.5 Changes in the number and size of mitochondria of human skeletal muscle after training. (From Keissling *et al.* 1971.)

area of the muscle mitochondria. This is associated with an up to two-fold increase in the activity of TCA cycle enzymes and components of the electron transport chain. For example, as shown in Fig. 8.5, there was a 120% increase in the number of mitochondria in the vastus lateralis muscle of humans following a 28-week endurance-training programme. Increases in mitochondrial size are not as great as increases in number. On average, human skeletal muscle mitochondria are 14–40% larger in endurance athletes compared with sedentary individuals. However, this is a specific response, occurring only in those muscles involved in the exercise training.

During training, changes in the activity of individual enzymes within the mitochondria appear to occur to a different extent. For example, when rats were trained by daily treadmill running, the cytochrome *c* content of the gastrocnemius muscle was elevated above control values by 102% (Holloszy *et al.* 1970), whereas the activity of various TCA cycle enzymes increased by 34–101% (Fig. 8.6). The activity of isocitrate dehydrogenase, the rate-limiting enzyme in the TCA cycle was increased by 90% after training. This suggests that a change in the mitochondrial composition, as well as an increase in the activities of the TCA and electron transport enzymes, occurs as a result of endurance training. An increased level of activity or concentration of enzymes involved in the TCA cycle and electron transport chain confers a greater capacity to generate ATP in the presence of oxygen. It was previously thought that this increased aerobic metabolic capacity was not utilized because the mitochondrial content was considered to be more than adequate (i.e. in excess of maximal needs), even in untrained muscle. However, recent evidence suggests

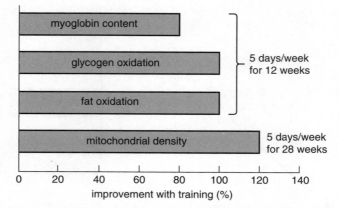

Fig. 8.6 Changes in enzyme activities and substrate oxidation capacities in rat skeletal muscle as a result of endurance training.

that an increase in mitochondrial content is needed to realize the increased potential for oxidative ATP supply induced in muscle by endurance training. These changes may be important in allowing the trained individual to sustain a higher percentage of aerobic capacity ($\dot{V}O_2$max) during prolonged exercise. The oxidative capacity of both the Type I and Type II fibres can be greatly enhanced by training; the increase in mitochondrial density is not specific to the Type I fibres. Indeed, in élite long-distance runners the capacity of Type II fibres to oxidize fuels, including lipid, may exceed the oxidative capacity of the Type I fibres of untrained individuals.

However, differential changes in the metabolic characteristics of the different fibre types can be induced by different types of training. One study found that both high-intensity interval training carried out at maximal intensity and continuous submaximal exercise resulted in increases in the muscle succinate dehydrogenase (SDH) activity of about 20–30%. Analysis of single fibres, however, showed that the high-intensity training programme had increased the SDH activity of Type II fibres by about 50% with no increase in the SDH activity in Type I fibres. The continuous-running training programme resulted in a 30% increase in the SDH activity of Type I fibres, with no change in the SDH activity of Type II fibres. An increased oxidative enzyme activity in the Type II fibres may be of primary importance for increasing endurance capacity by reducing the reliance of these fibres on anaerobic glycolysis for ATP production.

8.3 Modification of the metabolic response to exercise by endurance training

Changes in the metabolic response to an acute exercise bout following a programme of endurance training are summarized in Table 8.4. Trained muscle

Table 8.4   Modification of the metabolic response to exercise by endurance training

Lower RER and muscular RQ
Smaller rise in plasma free fatty acid concentration
Lower rate of utilization of muscle glycogen
Reduced utilization of blood glucose by muscle
Reduced accumulation of muscle lactate
Increase in oxidation of lipid relative to carbohydrate
Increased utilization of intramuscular triglyceride

exhibits a greater capability to oxidize carbohydrate. Consequently, large amounts of pyruvate can be converted to acetyl-CoA and moved through the TCA cycle. There is also an increase in the capacity of trained muscle to take up and oxidize lipid (Fig. 8.7). This occurs via the increased capillary density in muscle, allowing a greater surface area for FFA uptake from blood and an increase in the activity of lipid-mobilizing and lipid-metabolizing enzymes. The activity of lipoprotein lipase (LPL) in the capillary endothelium of trained muscle is increased and the capacity for β-oxidation of FFA within the mitochondria is enhanced. However, the major effect of the enzymatic changes which take place in muscle during endurance training is to increase the con-

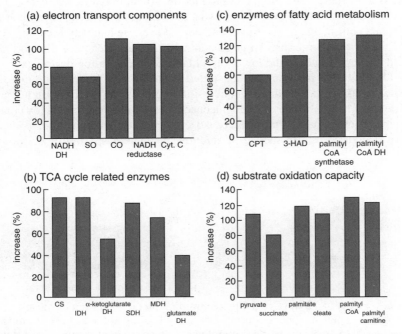

Fig. 8.7 The effects of training on the aerobic potential of skeletal muscle. See earlier Chapters for details of enzymes (From Holloszy 1973, Mole *et al.* 1971, and Kiessling *et al.* 1971.)

tribution of lipid, and correspondingly decrease the contribution of carbohydrate to oxidative energy metabolism (i.e. ATP production) during submaximal exercise. Numerous studies have confirmed that training lowers the respiratory exchange ratio (RER) during exercise and also (determined in invasive experiments) the local respiratory quotient (RQ) measured directly across the exercising limbs. This increased oxidation of lipid is probably a consequence of an increase in the potential for the oxidation of substrates relative to the glycolytic capacity, which appears to show a smaller adaptive response to endurance training. The endurance-trained athlete not only uses more fat and less carbohydrate at the same absolute exercise intensity, but also at the same relative exercise intensity expressed as a percentage of $\dot{V}O_2$max. Both the utilization of intramuscular glycogen and the oxidation of blood-borne glucose are decreased after training (Fig. 8.8). In cardiac muscle, this glycogen-sparing effect has been shown to be mediated by the operation of the glucose–fatty acid cycle, whereby an increased lipid oxidation results in intracellular citrate accumulation and the consequent inhibition of glycolysis at the level of phosphofructokinase, but there is some debate as to whether this mechanism operates in human skeletal muscle.

A reduction in the uptake and utilization of blood glucose by muscle also reduces the extent of liver glycogenolysis and contributes to the better maintenance of blood glucose homeostasis during prolonged exercise. Associated with the decreased rate of carbohydrate oxidation during exercise in the trained state is a decreased rate of lactate production. At submaximal exercise intensities, the trained individual has a lower blood lactate concentration than the untrained person; again this is true whether the exercise intensity is expressed in absolute or relative terms. An enhancement of lactate clearance after training could also contribute to the lower blood lactate concentration during exercise, and although this has been demonstrated in the rat it appears to be due to a greater uptake of lactate and its conversion to glucose by the liver. In humans, on the other hand, the rate of liver gluconeogenesis during exercise is lower after training. These two important effects, a decreased rate of carbohydrate oxidation and a decreased rate of lactate production, result in a sparing of the body's

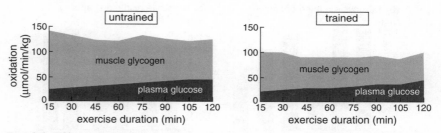

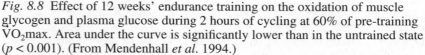

Fig. 8.8 Effect of 12 weeks' endurance training on the oxidation of muscle glycogen and plasma glucose during 2 hours of cycling at 60% of pre-training $\dot{V}O_2$max. Area under the curve is significantly lower than in the untrained state ($p < 0.001$). (From Mendenhall *et al.* 1994.)

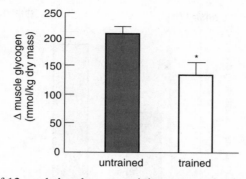

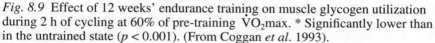

Fig. 8.9 Effect of 12 weeks' endurance training on muscle glycogen utilization during 2 h of cycling at 60% of pre-training $\dot{V}O_2$max. * Significantly lower than in the untrained state ($p < 0.001$). (From Coggan *et al.* 1993).

limited carbohydrate reserves: the rate of utilization of muscle glycogen is lower after training (Fig. 8.9). In view of the close link between the availability of muscle glycogen as a fuel and endurance capacity (see Chapters 3 and 7), this decreased rate of glycogen utilization is a major factor in improving performance in endurance events.

Alterations in substrate use with training could also be due to a lesser degree of disturbance to ATP homeostasis during exercise: with a greater mitochondrial capacity after training, smaller decreases in ATP and PCr and smaller increases in ADP and P_i are needed during exercise to balance the rate of ATP synthesis with the rate of ATP utilization. In other words, with more mitochondria, the oxygen as well as the ADP and P_i required per mitochondrion will be less after training compared with before training. The smaller increase in ADP concentration would result in less formation of AMP by the adenylate kinase reaction, and also less IMP and ammonia would be formed as a result of the AMP deaminase reaction. Smaller increases in intramuscular concentrations of AMP and P_i could account for the slower rate of glycogenolysis and glycolysis in trained compared with untrained muscle.

Clearly, the training-induced reduction in carbohydrate oxidation during exercise is compensated for by an increased rate of lipid oxidation. For many years this was assumed to be due to an increased muscle uptake and oxidation of plasma-borne FFA derived from lipolysis in adipose tissue. However, several well-controlled studies fail to support this notion and indicate that not only is plasma FFA concentration during exercise lower after training, but so is the uptake and oxidation of plasma FFA. An alternative source of the increased lipid oxidation after training may come from intramuscular triacylglycerol stores, and evidence in support of this has come from studies which have reported that training resulted in a much greater utilization of intramuscular triacylglycerol during prolonged exercise (Fig. 8.10). In one such study, the increased

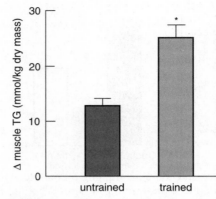

Fig. 8.10 Effect of 12 weeks' endurance training on muscle triglyceride utilization during 2-h of cycling at 60% of pre-training $\dot{V}O_2$max. * Significantly higher than in the untrained state ($p < 0.001$) (From Hurley *et al.* 1986.)

intramuscular lipolysis could have supplied all the additional fat oxidized after training, assuming that at least 8 kg of muscle was activated during the exercise.

The rate of hydrolysis of VLDL-triacylglycerol is also increased by training as a result of the increase in muscle LPL activity and greater capillary endothelial surface area following training. But even so, VLDL-triacylglycerols could not account for more than about 10% of total energy expenditure. This effect of training could, however, be partly responsible for the improvement in the blood lipid profile observed when previously sedentary subjects take up a more active lifestyle. Replenishment of intramuscular triacylglycerol stores after prolonged exercise may also improve the clearance of triacylglycerol from the blood.

8.4 Physiological adaptations to endurance training influencing the metabolic response to exercise

A consideration of the effects of endurance training on exercise metabolism would be incomplete if account was not taken of the central cardiovascular and respiratory adaptations to training that influence the delivery of oxygen to the working muscles. The capacity to perform endurance exercise depends on the maximum aerobic power that can be developed ($\dot{V}O_2$max) and on the fraction of $\dot{V}O_2$ max that can be sustained. In exercise involving a large muscle mass, such as running or cycling, the $\dot{V}O_2$max is most commonly limited by oxygen delivery to the working muscles rather than by the capacity of the muscles to extract and use oxygen. The peak stroke volume of the heart appears to be closely related to $\dot{V}O_2$max and to the changes in $\dot{V}O_2$max that occur with training and detraining. Peripheral factors, especially the increased capillary density in muscle and the increased oxidative capacity, as previously described, will allow for an increased utilization of lipid as a metabolic fuel during exercise and may be of particular importance for improving endurance capacity.

The main effects of endurance training on cardiovascular and respiratory function are briefly described below and summarized in Table 8.5, but for a more detailed description and discussion of the changes the reader is referred to several exercise physiology texts (see further reading list at the end of this chapter).

Élite endurance athletes can achieve a high $\dot{V}O_2$max and they also have the ability to exercise for prolonged periods at a high percentage of their $\dot{V}O_2$max. The physiological and metabolic factors which contribute to this ability have been extensively studied. To achieve a high rate of oxygen consumption, an effective system for the transfer (delivery) of oxygen from the atmosphere to the working muscles is required coupled with an effective extraction of oxygen from the blood flowing through the active musculature. In the absence of pulmonary disease, the first stage of this process, the transfer of oxygen from the atmospheric air to the blood passing through the pulmonary capillaries, is not a limiting factor. Virtually full oxygen saturation of haemoglobin in blood is achieved during maximal exercise, except possibly in elderly subjects or in athletes with an extremely high $\dot{V}O_2$max.

Table 8.5 Physiological adaptations to endurance training

Blood volume:	Increase in plasma volume and total haemoglobin
Stroke volume:	Increased due to an enlarged ventricular volume accompanied by enhanced myocardial contractility
Heart rate:	Decreased at rest and during submaximal exercise No change in maximum heart rate
Cardiac output:	Increased maximum cardiac output due to higher stroke volume
Blood flow and distribution:	Increased total muscle blood flow during maximal exercise. Reduced regional blood flow to working muscle during submaximal exercise
Oxygen extraction:	Increased extraction of oxygen from blood flowing through working muscle and hence an increase in the arteriovenous oxygen difference
Arterial blood pressure:	Reduced systolic and diastolic blood pressure at rest and during submaximal exercise
Ventilation:	Larger maximum lung ventilation rate due to increases in both tidal volume and breathing frequency. Lower ventilation rates during submaximal exercise

Whole body oxygen consumption can be described by the Fick equation:

$$\dot{V}O_2 = \quad \underset{\text{(beats min}^{-1})}{[\text{Heart rate}} \times \underset{\text{(litre beat}^{-1})}{\text{Stoke volume}]} \times \underset{\text{(ml O}_2 \text{ litre}^{-1})}{[\text{a–v oxygen difference}]}$$
$$(\text{ml O}_2 \text{ min}^{-1})$$

Stroke volume is the amount of blood ejected by the heart with each beat, and the product of the stroke volume and heart rate gives the cardiac output, that is to say the volume of blood pumped into the systemic circulation each minute. The arterio–venous (a–v) oxygen difference is the difference in oxygen content between arterial and mixed venous blood, and, therefore, represents the amount of oxygen extracted from the blood as it flows through the tissues.

The high maximum cardiac output achieved by endurance athletes depends on a higher than normal stroke volume. During maximal work the heart rate is usually no different (or slightly less) compared with that of untrained individuals. The high stroke volumes are achieved as a consequence of increased ventricular size, greater end-diastolic volume, and enhanced myocardial contractility. Cardiac output at rest is similar in well-trained and untrained individuals, and thus the higher stroke volume of the athlete is associated with a lower resting heart rate. During submaximal exercise, cardiac output may be lower after training as less blood flow is required to meet the muscle's oxygen needs (as extraction increases). During maximal exercise, endurance athletes also display a higher oxygen extraction from the blood despite the increased muscle blood flow rate.

The oxygen carrying capacity of the blood (namely the maximum arterial oxygen content) is determined largely by its haemoglobin content: each gram of haemoglobin can transport 1.34 ml oxygen when fully saturated. It seems somewhat surprising, therefore, that highly trained endurance athletes are commonly observed to have lower blood haemoglobin concentrations than their sedentary counterparts. However, this arises, at least in part, from an increase in the total blood volume, with a greater relative increase in plasma volume compared with the red cell mass (and hence a dilutional decrease in the red cell count per litre of blood). Even so, total blood haemoglobin content is increased in endurance athletes, and the decrease in blood haemoglobin concentration is compensated for by an increase in red cell 2,3-diphosphoglycerate (2,3-DPG) content. The ability of blood to deliver oxygen to the muscles is enhanced by 2,3-DPG as this compound (a glycolytic intermediate) reduces the affinity of haemoglobin for oxygen. The lower red cell count of the athlete's blood reduces the viscosity of the blood, reducing resistance to blood flow through the vasculature and reducing the work of the heart, which may have benefits in allowing increased blood flow during very intense exercise. Hence, there is conclusive evidence that the delivery of oxygen to the working muscles is increased as a result of endurance training. The increased availability of oxygen during exercise at high intensities, coupled with increased extraction in the trained state and the increased oxidative capacity of the muscle tissue allows a greater contribution to ATP production to be made from the oxidation of fatty acids.

8.5 Time course of endurance training adaptations and of detraining

The extent of adaptation to training is dependent mostly on the training load (namely intensity × duration × frequency of exercise) and is specific to the muscles recruited during the activity. Training must be performed for several weeks or months to allow the muscle-specific biochemical adaptations to reach a new steady state (Fig. 8.3). For mitochondrial content at least, exercise intensity interacts with the duration of the exercise bout; peak adaptations in mitochondrial content seem to occur with shorter durations of exercise as the intensity of each bout is increased from about 40% up to 90% $\dot{V}O_2$max. The proven benefit of prolonged training sessions in improving endurance performance may be more related to adaptations in cardiovascular function, blood volume, and fluid balance rather than to muscle-specific adaptations in oxidative capacity.

The time course of training-induced alterations in substrate utilization during exercise closely parallels the time course of the increase in mitochondrial enzyme activities in most long-term longitudinal exercise training studies, and a similar response is evident during detraining. However, recent studies have been unable to detect changes in mitochondrial enzyme activities or oxidative capacity after 5–7 days of training, although RER and muscle glycogen utilization during exercise were reduced compared with before training. It seems possible that in the early stages of training, mechanisms other than an increase in mitochondrial metabolic capacity are responsible for training-induced changes in substrate use during exercise. Other factors could include an early alteration in the hormonal response to exercise; there is evidence that the catecholamine response to exercise is significantly attenuated after only a few training bouts have been performed. For example, it has been reported that after just one week of training, there was a 40% drop an plasma adrenaline concentration and a 25% decrease in noradrenaline in response to submaximal exercise at 70% $\dot{V}O_2$max.

Maintenance of endurance-training adaptations can only be achieved by continuing to perform exercise on a regular basis. Training adaptations are lost during periods of inactivity (Fig. 8.3 and Fig. 8.11). Some variables can be lost within an alarmingly short time. For example, about 50% of the increased mitochondrial content induced by training can be lost within 1 month of detraining (Fig. 8.12). A return to training will, of course, allow recovery of the muscle adaptations, but the time required to re-establish the original trained condition can take somewhat longer than the detraining interval over which they were lost.

8.6 Hormonal adaptations to endurance training

The increase in muscle oxidative capacity is not the only way in which substrate metabolism is modified in response to training. Neuroendocrine responses play an important role in controlling the mobilization and utilization of fuel

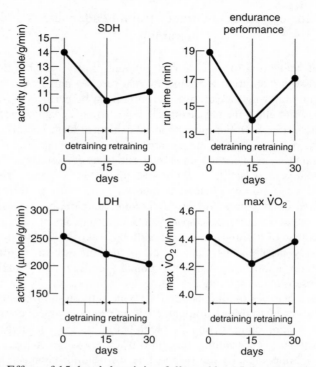

Fig. 8.11 Effect of 15 days' detraining followed by 15 days' retraining in six male competitive runners on muscle activities of succinate dehydrogenase (SDH) and lactate dehydrogenase (LDH), endurance performance and $\dot{V}O_2$max. Detraining induced significant falls in all variables by 15 days. The 15-day period of retraining did not return all the variables to their previous levels. (From Houston *et al.* 1979.)

substrates during exercise, particularly when the exercise duration lasts for more than a few minutes. In general, the hormonal responses to an exercise stress are significantly attenuated after training. For example, a smaller rise in the plasma concentration of adrenaline occurs during exercise at both the same absolute and relative exercise intensities in the trained state compared with before training. Sympathetic nervous activity, as reflected by the plasma noradrenaline concentration during exercise, is decreased at the same absolute work rate after training, but remains constant in relation to the same relative work rate. Adrenocorticotrophic hormone, cortisol, glucagon, and growth hormone levels also increase less during submaximal exercise in trained subjects. Insulin concentration usually falls during acute exercise. In trained subjects this decrease is less and, therefore, plasma insulin concentration tends to be higher in trained individuals during exercise. The smaller fall in plasma insulin during exercise after training may, in part, reflect the smaller degree of inhibition of insulin

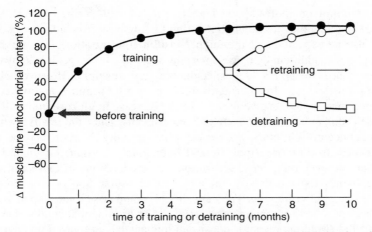

Fig. 8.12 Time course of training and detraining adaptations in mitochondrial density in skeletal muscle.

secretion by the diminished exercising adrenaline concentration. These training effects may be partly due to the increased $\dot{V}O_2$max with training, but this is not the only reason as the attenuation of most hormonal responses is also evident when trained individuals are exercised at the same relative exercise intensities as before training (or for sedentary controls). Furthermore, the effects of training are only evident when the same mode of exercise as used in the training programme is employed even though $\dot{V}O_2$max may be identical under different conditions. Also during the detraining of highly conditioned athletes over a number of weeks, during which $\dot{V}O_2$max falls, catecholamine responses to submaximal exercise are not altered. Hence, these adaptations in the hormonal response to exercise represent a specific response to training, and are not just an effect of the accompanying change in $\dot{V}O_2$max.

The physiological implications of some of these neuroendocrine adaptations to training are fairly clear. For example, the lower levels of cortisol and catecholamines would imply a lesser overall stress, and the lower heart rate that is also a feature of physical training can be explained, at least in part, by this decreased catecholamine response. Interpretation of the metabolic consequences of the hormonal changes accompanying training is more difficult.

The slower rate of muscle glycogenolysis during exercise after training could be due, in part, to lower adrenaline concentrations. The latter together with the attenuated decline in plasma insulin is also likely to contribute to the lower rate of liver glucose production and lower adipose tissue lipolysis during exercise after training. These conclusions generally assume no change in the tissue responsiveness to the hormone concerned, but this may not always be the case. For example, the lipolytic activity of the adipose depots of rats becomes more sensitive to the effects of adrenaline after physical training. Insulin, though, is a potent inhibitor of lipolysis, and higher insulin levels during exercise in the trained state may play a role in attenuating FFA release from adipose tissue. It might also be expected that this higher insulin concentration during exercise would promote additional glucose uptake by skeletal muscle, yet it is known that training reduces the uptake of plasma glucose during exercise. However, plasma insulin levels are quite low during exercise, even after training, and it has been estimated that, in humans, about 85% of the increase in glucose uptake during exercise is due to non-insulin mediated mechanisms. Thus, the relatively higher insulin concentration during exercise after training is probably of more significance in inhibiting lipolysis and liver glucose production than for its potential influence on glucose utilization by muscle. None of these endocrine changes can satisfactorily explain why intramuscular lipolysis is increased during exercise after training. Theoretically this could arise if the responsiveness of skeletal muscle to adrenaline was increased by training, but studies that have investigated β_2-adrenoreceptor density in humans have reported no change in response to endurance training. The fact that intramuscular glycogenolysis, which is also stimulated via β_2-adrenoreceptors, is relatively lower during exercise in the trained state also argues against a generalized increased skeletal muscle responsiveness to the actions of adrenaline.

8.7 Adaptation to sprint and strength training

Training for strength, power, or speed has little, if any, effect on aerobic capacity, and relatively little cardiovascular adaptation ensues. This is consistent with the principle of the specificity of training. Relatively brief bouts of heavy resistance exercise or sprinting, both of which demand a high level of anaerobic metabolism, bring about specific changes in the immediate (ATP and PCr) and short-term (glycolysis) energy delivery systems (Table 8.6) and an improvement in sprint performance. The latter includes an increase in the maximum power output, an increase in the amount of work done during a brief intense exercise bout of fixed duration, and an increase in exercise duration (endurance) at high exercise intensities. Anaerobic capacity can be estimated indirectly by measuring the accumulated oxygen deficit during a 2–3 min treadmill run to exhaus-

Table 8.6   Muscle adaptation to strength training

Hypertrophy of muscle fibres
Increased muscle cross-sectional area
Increased phosphocreatine and glycogen content
Increased glycolytic capacity
Increased strength and high-intensity exercise capacity
Decreased mitochondrial density
Improved muscle buffering capacity

tion. Such studies have found that sprint training (three sessions per week for 6 weeks) increases the anaerobic capacity of human subjects by 10%.

Short-term, high-intensity training has little, if any, effect on muscle fibre type composition. Only one study has reported a significant increase in Type II fibres (from 32 to 38%) and a decrease in Type I fibres (from 57 to 48%) following 6 weeks of sprint cycle training. Relatively few studies on the effects of sprint training have been conducted, but those that have been done indicate that a marked degree of muscle hypertrophy does not occur. This may be due to the short duration of such studies (6–8 weeks has been the norm). Hypertrophy of fibres (particularly Type II) is known to occur with longer periods of heavy resistance or weight training. The diameter of fibres from the muscles of weightlifters and body builders is greater than those from sedentary individuals. Longitudinal studies indicate that the cross-sectional area of Type II fibres can be increased by about 50% after several months of weight training. Animal experiments, in which muscle hypertrophy is induced by the surgical removal of a synergistic muscle, confirm the hypertrophy of individual fibres, but suggest that total fibre numbers within the adapted muscle are unchanged. Postmortem investigation of the muscles of strength-trained athletes also indicates that such individuals do not have more muscle fibres than ordinary people.

Muscle biopsies taken before and after resistance training which increased muscular strength by 28%, indicate that resting intramuscular concentrations of ATP, PCr, and glycogen are increased by about 5, 10, and 10–30%, respectively. However, these measurements are the average concentrations from muscle sample homogenates, and may simply reflect the relative increase in Type II fibre area since, at rest, these fibres have been reported to have higher phosphagen and glycogen concentrations than the Type I fibres. Several studies have found no changes in resting intramuscular ATP and PCr concentrations after 4–8 weeks of sprint training, and this type of training did not induce significant muscle hypertrophy. The muscle glycogen store also increases after sprint training, which is not surprising given the importance of glycogen as a fuel in exercise involving repeated bouts of sprinting.

When sprint-running performance is improved as a result of sprint training, the rate of ATP turnover is further increased by an increased contribution from anaerobic glycolysis to the ATP supply. The amount and activity of enzymes involved in the glycolytic pathway (e.g. phosphofructokinase) has consistently been reported to increase with both sprint and weight training (Fig. 8.13), with the most dramatic changes occurring in the Type II fibres. However, the magnitude of these changes is not as great as that seen with the oxidative enzymes in response to aerobic endurance training. For example, one study reported that LDH activity of the vastus lateralis of élite weightlifters was 62% higher in Type II fibres compared with sedentary men; the activity of this enzyme was 50% higher in the Type I fibres of the weightlifters compared to the controls. Myokinase activity in the Type I fibres was no different, whereas in the Type II fibres it was 40% higher in the weight-trained athletes. With respect to changes

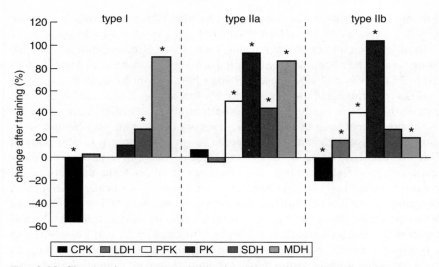

Fig. 8.13 Changes in enzyme activities in different fibre types following sprint training. * Significant change with training ($p < 0.05$). (From Takekura and Yoshioka 1990.)

in aerobic (mitochondrial) enzymes it has generally been found that where a significant hypertrophy of the fibres occurs, there is a reduction in activity of oxidative enzymes and cytochromes, which presumably reflects an increase in fibre cross-sectional area (primarily Type II) without an adaptive increase in mitochondrial content (that is to say a dilutional effect on mitochondrial density). The number of capillaries may remain unchanged in strength training, but the capillaries are more spaced out between larger muscle fibres resulting in a decreased capillary density per unit area (Fig. 8.1).

After anaerobic training, higher concentrations of lactate in the blood can be achieved during maximal exercise, which is probably due to the higher levels of intramuscular glycogen and glycolytic enzymes present after training. Heavy anaerobic training requires considerable motivation, and an improved level of motivation and pain tolerance to the metabolic acidosis accumulated may contribute to the higher levels of blood lactate seen after exercise in the anaerobically trained state. Improvements in the capacity of muscle to buffer the protons associated with lactate accumulation could also be important. Type II fibres have a higher buffering capacity and, therefore, growth of these fibres relative to Type I fibres would indicate an increase in muscle buffering capacity. Although there is little evidence for major increases in muscle physicochemical buffering as determined by titration after training, it appears that if buffering is calculated based on postexercise pH and lactate content, then buffering capacity is seen to rise with sprint training. The two components of buffering not determined by the titration method are the contributions of bicarbonate (the primary buffer in the extracellular fluid) and transmembrane hydrogen ion fluxes. The latter may provide an explanation for the finding of Nevill *et al.* (1989) that the post-exercise muscle physicochemical component of buffering and the postexercise muscle pH were the same before and after sprint training, even though the postexercise muscle lactate content was approximately 20% higher after training.

Improvements in muscular strength, at least during the first few weeks of a strength-training programme, are due to neural facilitation (disinhibition) leading to a full activation of motor units and muscle groups, since the early and rapid strength increases observed at the start of a training regimen are not associated with an increase in muscle size and cross-sectional area.

Longer term, heavy-resistance training results in muscle hypertrophy and further gains in strength. Improvements in strength are important since this results in the muscle working at a lower fraction of its maximum capability for force output when required to perform work. Increases in muscle mass mean that more muscle tissue is available to perform work, resulting in a greater peak power output and also a greater total capacity of the anaerobic energy-producing systems. The precise physiological and biochemical changes which take place in the muscle to produce these effects are not, at present, clear. Although the response to aerobic endurance training has been extensively studied in the laboratory, relatively little attention has been devoted to the study of the responses to anaerobic training.

It must be remembered, of course, that these effects are specific to the muscles used in the training programme, and more particularly to the individual muscle fibre types that are recruited during the exercise. It is apparent that very high-intensity training is necessary to activate the Type IIb fibres. At present, not enough evidence is available for sports scientists to make detailed recommendations regarding the intensity, frequency, and duration of training that will optimize the adaptive response.

8.8 Mechanisms of muscular adaptations to training

Two fundamental questions arise from the preceding description of how muscles adapt to training. One is; What is the precise nature of the stimulus (or stimuli) that induce(s) adaptation? The other is; What are the molecular mechanisms that allow such adaptation to occur? Answers to these questions are beginning to emerge from recent advances in molecular biology now being applied to skeletal muscle, investigating how this extremely plastic tissue adapts to increased use and disuse. Whilst an in-depth review of this topic is beyond the scope of this book, a brief summary of recent research findings is given below.

It seems certain that the myosin gene family holds the key to muscle plasticity. There are at least seven different versions available, so the muscle fibres are inherently flexible. In theory, they can alter their contractile properties by rebuilding their myofibrils using a different type of myosin heavy chain. A fast-twitch muscle fibre could become a slow fibre simply by switching off the gene for the fast-myosin heavy chain and switching on the gene for the slow isoform of the protein. Most genes in the cells of the body are switched on and off by the indirect actions of signalling molecules such as hormones or growth factors. Adaptations in muscle in response to training are specific to the muscles used in the activity; unused muscles do not adapt. Thus, it seems that muscle genes are regulated largely by mechanical and/or metabolic stimuli. It is the stretching or contracting of a muscle fibre which turns specific genes on or off. The activity of different myosin genes can be monitored using DNA probes. Animal experiments have elegantly demonstrated that stretch alone and contraction alone (induced by electrical stimulation) in a fast muscle (e.g. tibialis anterior) only slightly affected the activities of myosin genes. However, together these stimuli caused a dramatic shutdown in the synthesis of the fast-myosin heavy chain, switching almost exclusively to the slow version of myosin. Immobilization of a slow muscle (soleus) in the rabbit caused the muscle to revert to expressing the fast-myosin gene. Thus, it appears that the fast myosin is the 'default option'. A slow muscle, such as the soleus, needs to be repeatedly stretched to sustain its synthesis of the slow-myosin heavy chain. Both these observations are consistent with what we know about the effects of different types of training regimens on human muscles.

Stretching the muscle fibres during exercise is one potent stimulus to adaptation. Passive stretch is known to induce muscle enlargement even in the absence of innervation, insulin, growth hormone, or adequate nutrition. The transduction of mechanical forces through the cytoskeleton to the nuclei and polyribosomes of the muscle fibres may occur either directly or via membrane-bound, stretch-activated ion channels or stretch-induced alterations in plasma membrane-associated molecules (e.g. mechanoresponsive isoforms of adenylate cyclase). These stretch-related signals could then induce altered gene expression (e.g. of muscle growth factors) and altered rates of protein synthesis and degradation.

Either increased cAMP levels or the rate of metabolic flux is hypothesized to be the signal for increased mitochondrial biogenesis resulting from endurance-type training. A relationship has been found between increases in adenylate cyclase activity, intracellular cAMP concentration, and mRNA molecules for mitochondrial proteins during the continuous electrical stimulation of skeletal muscle. Increased metabolic flux could be signalled via an increase in the ADP/ATP ratio or a decrease in phosphocreatine.

Damage to muscle fibres during exercise may also provide a stimulus for adaptation. High concentrations of a muscle-specific growth factor released from damaged, degenerating (necrotic) muscle fibres, together with the loss of contact inhibition between satellite cells and underlying live muscle fibres, commit satellite cells to proliferation during the first day after muscle injury. Exercise-induced alteration of muscle Z-lines, cytoskeleton, or the extracellular matrix may, therefore, be obligatory for satellite-cell proliferation and fusion resulting in hypertrophy. The newly recruited satellite cells must provide the additional nuclei required to maintain nuclear density in hypertrophied muscle. A number of DNA hybridization studies have demonstrated a derepression of a muscle regulatory factor in muscle fibre nuclei during muscle regeneration and a localization of myosin heavy-chain mRNA in focal areas of damage produced in overstretched muscle.

Changes in the expression of the different myosin isoforms (and isoforms of the other contractile proteins) occur during apparent transformations of fibre types induced by cross-innervation of muscles (surgical intervention), chronic electrical stimulation, and disuse atrophy. Levels of thyroid hormones and growth hormone have been shown to influence such changes in myosin heavy-chain isoforms in skeletal muscle experiencing altered contractile activity. Muscle-specific protein adaptations show a sequential appearance of alterations in groups of proteins. For example, specific gene groups appear to respond in the following order: Ca^{2+}-handling proteins change first, followed by mitochondrial proteins, and contractile proteins are altered last. The same order of change in gene sets seems to occur in both the slow-to-fast conversion of postural muscles induced by relief from weight-bearing activity, and the conversion of fast to slow muscle which can be induced by prolonged electrical stimulation.

8.9 Training adaptations in blood lipid levels

Several training studies have shown that regular endurance exercise causes decreases in total blood cholesterol, triacylglycerol, and LDL concentrations and an increase in HDL concentration (Fig. 8.14). As mentioned in Chapter 4, HDL-cholesterol is thought to be protective against the development of atherosclerotic plaques and coronary artery disease, whereas a high level of LDL-cholesterol predisposes the individual to these conditions. Clearly, other factors such as smoking, diet, alcohol intake, family history, and other conditions such as obesity and diabetes are also important, and not all exercise intervention studies have established a clear independent relationship between exercise and fitness and blood lipids. In general, the available data suggest that individuals who have a high level of plasma cholesterol, LDL, and triacylglycerol levels will experience favourable changes in these variables after endurance type training. Large cross-sectional studies indicate an inverse relationship between cardiorespiratory fitness (endurance time or $\dot{V}O_2$max) and fasting serum or plasma triacylglycerol concentration, but there is no apparent relationship with muscular strength, suggesting that heavy-resistance training might not be associated with similar potential health benefits.

Endurance-trained individuals show characteristically high rates of triacylglycerol clearance from plasma compared with sedentary controls. These may be related to the increase in muscle LPL activity and muscle capillary density with training which might be expected to increase the rate of clearance

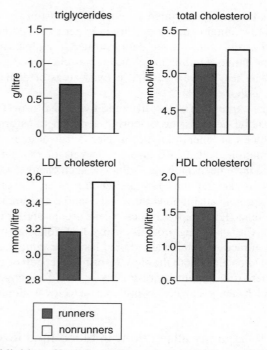

Fig. 8.14 Blood lipid profiles of middle-aged men who were either inactive or who ran an average of 39 miles (62 km) per week. (From Wood *et al.* 1976.)

of VLDL-triacylglycerol from the circulation. Rates of triacylglycerol degradation are closely coupled with rates of HDL synthesis, and so an enhanced metabolic capacity for triacylglycerol metabolism may explain the higher plasma HDL-cholesterol levels in exercise-trained people. During recovery from prolonged intense exercise (e.g. marathon running) fasting serum triacylglycerol concentrations are reduced and triacylglycerol clearance rates are increased. Recent studies indicate that less intense exercise (uphill walking) reduces the lipaemic response to a fatty meal either when the exercise is performed some hours before or some hours after the meal. The effect of exercise is greater after exercise at 60% $\dot{V}O_2$max than after a comparable duration of exercise at 30% $\dot{V}O_2$max, but this appears to be due to the greater overall energy expenditure rather than to the exercise intensity itself. An additional energy expenditure of about 3 MJ is required to attenuate the increase in blood triacylglycerol concentration following a fatty meal consumed 16 h later, and this effect appears to be greater in trained individuals. This effect could possibly be due to an enhanced clearance of triacylglycerol from the circulation for the purpose of restoring intramuscular triacylglycerol stores used during the exercise bout.

8.10 Immunosuppression associated with heavy training

Athletes engaged in heavy training programmes, particularly those involved in endurance events, appear to be more susceptible to infection. For example, sore throats and flu-like symptoms are more common in athletes than in the general population, and once infected, colds may last longer in athletes. There is some convincing evidence that this increased susceptibility to infection arises from a depression of immune system function.

The main component of the immune system comprises the white blood cells (leucocytes), whose numbers and functional capacities may be decreased by repeated bouts of intense prolonged exercise. The reason why immune function can be deleteriously affected by exercise is still unclear, but is probably related to increased levels of stress hormones during exercise. Some very recent research suggests that falls in the blood concentration of glutamine, an amino acid essential for the optimal functioning of leucocytes, may also be implicated in causing the immunosuppression associated with heavy training. Muscle damage may also be a factor.

An acute bout of physical activity is accompanied by responses that are remarkably similar in many respects to those induced by infection: there is a substantial increase in the number of circulating leucocytes (mainly lympho-cytes and neutrophils), the magnitude of which is related to both the intensity and duration of exercise. There are also increases in the plasma concentrations of various substances that are known to influence leucocyte functions, including tumour necrosis factor, interleukins 1, 2, and 6, acute-phase proteins like C-reactive protein, and activated complement fragments. Hormonal changes also occur in response to exercise, including rises in the plasma concentration of several hormones (e.g. adrenaline, cortisol, growth hormone, and prolactin) that are known to have immunomodulatory effects. Acute exercise temporarily increases the phagocytic activity of neutrophils and macrophages and increases natural killer (NK) cell lytic activity, but it has been shown to diminish the proliferative response of lymphocytes to mitogens.

During recovery from exercise, NK cell numbers and activity fall below pre-exercise levels, and if the exercise bout was of high intensity, the number of circulating lymphocytes may be decreased below pre-exercise levels for several hours after exercise and the T-lymphocyte CD4+/CD8+ (helper/suppressor) ratio is decreased. Following long-term intense exercise the production of immunoglobulins (antibodies) by B lymphocytes is inhibited. These changes during early recovery from exercise would appear to weaken the potential immune response to pathogens and they have been suggested to provide an 'open window' for infection representing the most vulnerable time period for an athlete in terms of their susceptibility to contracting an infection.

Exercise training also modifies immune function, with most changes, on balance, suggesting an overall decrease in immune system function, particularly when training loads are high. The circulating numbers of leucocytes are generally lower in athletes at rest compared with sedentary people, and increases in the leucocyte count during exercise (at the same absolute or relative intensity) are lower after training. The phagocytic activity of blood neutrophils has been reported to be markedly lower in trained cyclists compared with age and weight-matched sedentary controls. Levels of secretory immunoglobulins, such as salivary IgA, are lower in well-trained subjects, as are T-lymphocyte CD4+/CD8+ ratios and *in vitro* mitogen-stimulated, lymphocyte proliferation responses.

There are several possible causes of the diminution of immune function associated with heavy training. One mechanism may simply be the cumulative effects of repeated bouts of intense exercise with the consequent elevation of stress hormones, particularly glucocorticoids, causing temporary immunosuppression; when exercise is repeated frequently there may be insufficient time for the immune system to fully recover. Furthermore, following exercise-induced muscle damage, plasma cortisol levels can be chronically elevated for several days.

Plasma glutamine levels can change substantially after exercise and may become severely depressed after high-intensity interval training. Repeated bouts of high-intensity training sessions appear to induce a sustained fall in the plasma glutamine concentration. Glutamine is essential for several functions of white blood cells including their ability to undergo cell division, to produce antibodies, and to destroy bacteria by ingestion and digestion. Skeletal muscle is thought to be the main source of glutamine released into the bloodstream and this release may play an important role in delivering glutamine to the cells of the immune system. In addition to exercise, other forms of stress such as trauma, surgery, and infection are known to cause an increased release of glutamine from skeletal muscle, to increase glutamine requirements by other organs, and to decrease plasma glutamine levels, which may account for the impaired immune function associated with these stress states.

Complement activation also occurs during exercise, and a diminution of the serum complement concentration with repeated bouts of exercise, particularly when muscle damage is incurred, could also contribute to decreased non-specific immunity in athletes; well-trained individuals have a lower serum complement concentration compared with sedentary controls.

8.11 Overtraining

Athletes can suffer from overtraining, a condition in which under-performance is experienced despite continued or even increased training. Although improvements in athletic performance hinge on increasing the training load or 'overloading', overtraining—a vicious circle of more training producing lower performance and chronic fatigue—seems to be a stress response to training too hard too often, with insufficient recovery time between exercise bouts.

The reasons why some athletes become overtrained while others do not is unclear, and the consequences range from altered muscle function to motivation. The pathophysiology of overtraining can include muscle soreness and weakness, cytokine actions, hormonal and haematological changes, mood swings and psychological depression, and nutritional problems such as loss of appetite and diarrhoea. In some cases the underlying cause could be a persistent viral infection, similar to glandular fever; several types of virus are known to infiltrate skeletal and cardiac muscle. A marked fall in the blood leucocyte count is often indicative of a chronic viral infection. Athletes suffering from the overtraining syndrome are also often reported to be immunosuppressed. Plasma glutamine could also be implicated here, as some studies have reported that overtrained athletes have low plasma glutamine levels, even in the resting state, and that these can remain low for several weeks, with recovery only taking place when the training load was markedly reduced. Alternatively, declines in plasma glutamine concentration may be caused by an infection: falls in plasma glutamine concentration have been observed in humans following exposure to viral stress.

The under-performance may be the result of exercise-induced muscle damage—many athletes who have been diagnosed as suffering from overtraining have reported that their muscles feel sore—which causes a loss of muscle strength. The consequences of exercise-induced muscle damage include: muscle pain, soreness, and stiffness; a reduced range of motion; a higher than normal blood lactate concentration and perceived exertion during exercise; a loss of strength, and reduced maximal dynamic power output that can last 5–10 days.

A practical index of muscle damage in athletes performing heavy training is the elevation of muscle proteins (e.g. myoglobin, creating kinase, lactate dehydrogenase, and myosin heavy-chain fragments) in the blood plasma. The damaged muscle tissue can cause an initial activation of the immune system, as white blood cells are attracted to the damaged muscles to begin the breakdown of damaged muscle fibres and initiate the repair process. However, increased levels of stress hormones such as cortisol also appear in the blood and these can have quite a potent depressing effect on the white blood cells. While this might be seen as the body's natural response to prevent excessive damage of the muscles by the immune system, it may also weaken the immune response to invading bacteria and viruses, rendering the unfortunate athlete more susceptible to infection.

Another detrimental effect of exercise-induced muscle damage is that it impairs the restoration of muscle glycogen stores. Glycogen becomes depleted after prolonged exercise. Damaged muscle has an impaired ability to take up glucose from the blood which is required to resynthesize glycogen in the muscle. This would be expected to result in a decreased endurance performance in subsequent exercise bouts.

Low, muscle glycogen stores induced by a combination of exercise and a diet low in carbohydrate have also been associated with falls in the intramuscular and plasma concentrations of glutamine, the amino acid mentioned previously, which is needed by leucocytes to enable them to carry out their functions of destroying bacteria and viruses. Thus, exercise-induced muscle damage could be expected to result in decreased athletic performance and make the athlete more prone to infection.

Dietary glutamine supplementation may improve the recovery of leucocyte function from exercise-induced induced stress and overtraining. Prolonged exercise, fasting, low carbohydrate diets, infection, and physical trauma (e.g. surgery) are all associated with falls in the plasma glutamine concentration. After surgery the intravenous infusion of glutamine, corresponding to about 0.2 g glutamine kg body mass^{-1} 24 h^{-1} preserves plasma and muscle glutamine concentration and diminishes the postoperative decline in skeletal muscle protein synthesis. Glutamine can also be taken orally and as a 1.5% w/v aqueous solution is almost tasteless. Consumption of such glutamine drinks can raise the plasma glutamine concentration substantially for several hours, and so could be consumed by athletes during or after exercise in order to prevent falls in the plasma glutamine concentration.

Adequate dietary intakes of micronutrients are important to preserve the immune system status. Deficiencies of vitamins A, B6, and C or of minerals including zinc and iron are known to be associated with the impairment of immunity. However, excessive doses can be harmful. Russian scientists have reported that the consumption of a plant extract (*Eleutherococcus senticosus*, ES) reduces the incidence of infection, and German scientists have reported that ES increases the circulating numbers of lymphocytes and NK cells in healthy normal subjects. The mechanism of action is not yet resolved, but may be due to ES-stimulated interferon production or macrophage activity: polysaccharides in ES may act as non-specific immune stimulants. Further well-controlled studies are required to establish if ES, glutamine, or zinc supplements could be used to bolster the immune system in athletes.

8.12 Key points

1. Several principles govern the nature and extent of physiological and metabolic adaptations to training. These include the overload principle, the specificity of exercise principle, and the reversibility principle.

2. Adaptations to aerobic endurance training include increases in capillary density, as well as mitochondrial size and number in trained muscle. The activity of TCA cycle and other oxidative enzymes are increased with a concomitant increase in the capacity to oxidize both lipid and carbohydrate.

3. Intramuscular stores of myoglobin, glycogen, and triacylglycerol are increased by endurance training.

4. Endurance training also brings about cardiovascular adaptations including enhanced blood volume, stroke volume and cardiac output, and an expanded arterio–venous oxygen difference.

5. During exercise, endurance-trained muscle exhibits lower rates of carbohydrate utilization and lactate production, whereas lipid oxidation rates are increased compared with untrained muscle. The main source of the increased lipid oxidation after training appears to be from intramuscular triacylglycerol.

6. Endurance training attenuates the magnitude of the hormonal responses to acute exercise.

7. Training for strength, power, or speed has little, if any, effect on aerobic capacity. Heavy resistance training or sprinting bring about specific changes in the immediate (ATP and PCr) and short-term (glycolytic) energy delivery systems, and improvements in strength and/or sprint performance.

8. Heavy resistance training for several months causes hypertrophy of the muscle fibres, thus increasing total muscle mass and the maximum power output that can be developed.

9. Stretch, contraction, and damage of muscle fibres during exercise provide the stimuli for adaptation, which involves changes in the expression of different myosin isoforms.

10. Heavy training loads appear to increase the susceptibility of the athlete to infections due to a diminution of immune system function.

Further reading

Astrand, P.-O. and Rodahl, K. (1986). *Textbook of work physiology*, (3rd ed). McGraw-Hill, New York.

Coggan, A. R. and Williams, B. D. (1995). Metabolic adaptations to endurance training: substrate metabolism during exercise. In: *Exercise metabolism* (ed. M. Hargreaves), pp. 177–210. Human Kinetics, Champaign, IL.

Fox, E. I., Bowers, R. W., and Foss, M. L. (1993). *The physiological basis for exercise and sport* (5th ed). WC Brown, Dubuque, IA.

Goldspink, G. (1992). The brains behind the brawn. *New Scientist* (1st August 1992), 28–33.

Powers, S. K. and Howley, E. T. (1990). *Exercise physiology. Theory and application to fitness and performance*, WC Brown, Dubuque, IA.

Saltin, B. Nazar, K., Costill, D. L., Stein, E., Jansson, E., Essen, B., *et al.* (1976). The nature of the training response; peripheral and central adaptations to one-legged exercise. *Acta Physiol. Scand.*, **96**, 289–305.

References

Andersen, P. and Henriksson, J. (1977). Training induced changes in the subgroups of human Type II skeletal muscle fibres. *Acta Physiol. Scand.*, **99**, 123–5.

Coggan, A. R., Spiner, R. J., Kohrt, W. M., and Holloszy, J. O. (1993). Effect of prolonged exercise on muscle citrate concentration before and after endurance training in men. *Am. J. Physiol.*, **275**, E215–E220.

Costill, D. L., Daniels, J., Evans, W., Fink, W., Krahenbuhl, G., and Saltin, B. (1976). Skeletal muscle enzymes and fiber composition in male and female track athletes. *J. Appl. Physiol.*, **40**, 149–54.

Henriksson, J., Chi, M. M.-Y., Hintz, C. S., Young, D. A., Kaiser, K. K., Salmons, S., *et al.* (1986). Chronic stimulation of mammalian muscle: changes in enzymes of six metabolic pathways. *Am. J. Physiol.*, **251**, C614–C632.

Holloszy, J. O. (1973). Biochemical adaptations to exercise: aerobic metabolism. *Exerc. Sports Sci. Rey.*, **1**, 45–71.

Holloszy, J. O., Oscai, L. B., Don, L. J., and Mole, P. A. (1970). Mitochondrial citric acid cycle and related enzymes: adaptive response to exercise. *Biochem. Biophys. Res. Commun.*, **40**, 1368–73.

Houston, M. E., Bentzen, H., and Larsen, H. (1979). Interrelationships between skeletal muscle adaptations and performance as studied by detraining and retraining. *Acta Physiol. Scand.*, **105**, 163–70.

Hurley, B. F., Nemeth, P. M., Martin, W. H., Hagberg, J. M., Dalsky, G. P., and Holloszy, J. O. (1986). Muscle triglyceride utilization during exercise: effect of training. *J. Appl. Physiol.*, **60**, 562–7.

Ingjer, F. (1979). Effects of endurance training on muscle fibre ATPase activity, capillary supply and mitochondrial content in man. *J. Physiol.*, **294**, 419–32.

Kiessling, K., Piehl, K., and Lundquist, C. (1971). Effect of physical training on ultrastructural features in human skeletal muscle. In: *Muscle metabolism during exercise* (ed. B. Pernow and B-Saltin). pp. 97–101. Plenum Press, New York.

Mendenhall, L. A., Swanson, S. C., Habash, D. L., and Coggan, A. R. (1994). Ten days of exercise training reduces glucose production and utilization during moderate-intensity exercise. *Am. J. Physiol.*, **266**, E136–E143.

Mole, P. A., Oscai, L. B., and Holloszy, J. O. (1971). Adaptation of muscle to exercise. Increase in levels of palmityl CoA synthetase, carnitine palmityl transferase, and palmityl CoA dehydrogenase, and the capacity to oxidise fatty acids. *J. Clin. Invest.*, **50**, 2323–30.

Nevill, M. E., Boobis, L. H., Brooks, S., and Williams, C. (1989). Effect of training on muscle metabolism during treadmill sprinting. *J. Appl. Physiol.*, **67**, 2376–82.

Simoneau, J.-A., Lortie, G., Boulay, M. R., Marcotte, M., Thibault, M.-C., and Bouchard, C. (1985). Human skeletal muscle fibre alteration with high-intensity intermittent training. *Eur. J. Appl. Physiol.*, **54**, 250–3.

Takekura, H. and Yoshioka, T. (1990). Different metabolic responses to exercise training programmes in single rat muscle fibers. *J. Muscle Res. Cell. Motil.*, **11**, 105–13.

Tesch, P. A., Thorsson, A., and Kaiser, P. (1984). Muscle capillary supply and fiber type characteristics in weight and power lifters. *J. Appl. Physiol.*, **56**, 35–8.

Wood, P. D., Haskell, W., Klein, H., Lewis, S., Stern, M. P., and Farquhar, J. W. (1976). The distribution of plasma lipoproteins in middle-aged male runners. *Metabolism*, **25**, 1249–57.

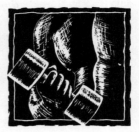

Appendix 1
Chemical structure and bonding

A1.1 Chemical structure

Although the distribution of electrical charges in chemical bonds is conveniently represented as being an all-or-nothing phenomenon, this is not in fact true: oxygen, for example, is more electronegative than carbon, and the electrons in a carbon–oxygen double bond will spend relatively more time in the vicinity of the oxygen atom than the carbon. Where a carboxyl group is present in a molecule, this leads to a slight negative charge on the oxygen and a corresponding positive charge on the carbon. These partial charge distributions are not the full charges that occur on ionization. They do, however, change the shape and charge distribution of the molecule, making it more or less susceptible to reaction with other charged molecules.

Many molecules can exist in more than one form, with the extremes of charge distribution being represented as distinct resonance or canonical forms, with the true structure being somewhere between these extremes.

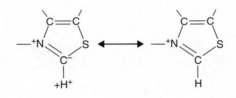

A1.1.1 Constitutional isomers

Even with the same chemical composition, different arrangements of the atoms within a molecule can give rise to entities with different chemical and physical properties. Compounds with identical molecular formulae, but with differences in the nature or sequence of their chemical bonds, or with differences in the spatial arrangements of their atoms are referred to as isomers, and a number of different forms of isomerism are possible. The nature and sequence of atoms in a molecule define its constitution, and molecules with the same components but different constitutions are referred to as constitutional isomers (formerly known as structural isomers). The amino acids leucine and isoleucine represent different arrangements of the same atoms to give distinct compounds:

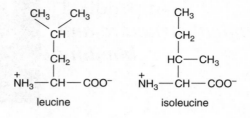

leucine   isoleucine

Glucose 6-phosphate and glucose 1-phosphate are isomers which are inter-converted by the enzyme phosphoglucomutase:

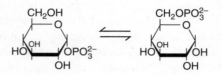

α-D-glucose 1-phosphate   α-D-glucose 6-phosphate

The bases which make up the structure of DNA can also exist in distinct chemical forms, or tautomers, with the proportions of the two forms being influenced by the pH of the local environment. This internal re-organization again results in an altered susceptibility to chemical reaction. An example is the structure of thymine:

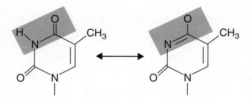

A1.1.2 Geometric stereoisomers

Geometric stereoisomers exist because of the different possible arrangements of chemical groups in relation to the double bonds in a molecule. Isomers are termed stereoisomers when the differ only in the arrangement of their atoms in space. Fumaric and maleic acid have the same component atoms, but in fumaric acid (the *trans* isomer) the carboxyl groups are effectively on opposite sides of the molecule, whereas in maleic acid (the *cis* isomer) the two carboxyl groups are both present on the same side of the molecule:

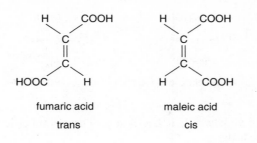

fumaric acid

trans

maleic acid

cis

A1.1.3 Optical stereoisomers

Whereas structural isomers and geometric stereoisomers have different chemical properties, optical stereoisomers are chemically identical in most respects, but they can be distinguished by one characteristic physical property. This is the characteristic rotation of the plane of polarized light falling on the molecule, either rotation to the right (dextrarotatory, d or + form) or to the left (laevorotatory, 1 or − form). This effect occurs because of the asymmetrical structure imposed on the carbon atom when it forms bonds with different groups. Glyceraldehyde is a relatively simple molecule that displays stereoisomerism. The D form is conventionally identified as having the hydroxyl group to the right and is dextrorotatory: the L form has the hydroxyl group to the left and is laevorotatory:

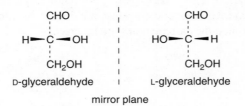

D-glyceraldehyde

mirror plane

L-glyceraldehyde

Each of the two possible structures is termed an enantiomer: if both forms are present in equal amounts, referred to as a racemic mixture, the effects cancel out and the mixture has no effect on polarized light.

The nomenclature becomes confusing when applied to other molecules. L-alanine is the enantiomer of alanine which corresponds to L-glyceraldehyde, and is the biologically important form: it is, however dextrorotatory, even though the corresponding form of glyceraldehyde is laevorotatory, and thus must be designated L-(+)-alanine.

To overcome this cumbersome and potentially ambiguous system of nomenclature, the R/S system has been adopted by the International Union of Biochemistry and Molecular Biology. This allocates to each sequential asymmetric carbon atom a symbol (R or S) depending on the arrangement of the

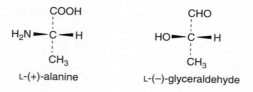

COOH   CHO

H_2N—C—H   HO—C—H

CH$_3$ CH$_3$

L-(+)-alanine   L-(–)-glyceraldehyde

groups or atoms with which it has bonds. The asymmetric carbon atom in D-glyceraldehyde is designated R.

A1.2 Structures of sugar molecules

A large number of different monosaccharides play an important role in metabolism as well as having structural and other roles. Monosaccharides are classified according to the number of carbon atoms present, with three (triose), five (pentose), and six (hexose) carbon molecules being of particular importance. Aldoses are sugars with an aldehyde group at the first carbon (and thus with structural similarity to glyceraldehyde), and ketoses have a ketone group (as in dihydroxyacetone): these two compounds, in their phosphorylated forms will be recognized as the products resulting from the action of aldolase on fructose 1,6-diphosphate.

Because of the large number of asymmetric carbon atoms in the pentoses and hexoses, many stereoisomers are possible, although only a few of these are biologically important. Glucose and galactose are diastereoisomers as not all of the configurations around the carbon atoms are reversed:

CHO   CH$_2$OH

HCOH   C=O

CH$_2$OH   CH$_2$OH

D-glyceraldehyde   dihydroxyacetone

CHO   CH$_2$OH

HCOH   C=O

HOCH   HOCH

HCOH   HCOH

HCOH   HCOH

CH$_2$OH   CH$_2$OH

D-glucose   D-fructose

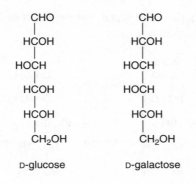

D-glucose   D-galactose

Pentoses and hexoses possess aldehyde and hydroxyl groups which can react with each other resulting in a molecule with a ring structure. The structure of glucose can, therefore, be represented as a linear molecule or as one of two possible (α and β) ring arrangements of the glucose atoms. The six-member ring of the hexoses consists of five carbon atoms and one oxygen atom:

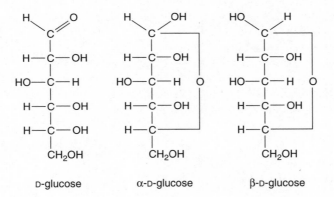

D-glucose α-D-glucose β-D-glucose

The ring structure of glucose is more usually represented as shown below for α-glucose 6-phosphate:

In the glucose phosphate isomerase reaction which catalyses the conversion of glucose 6-phosphate to fructose 6-phosphate, the ring structure must first be

broken to allow the reaction to proceed, but the fructose 6-phosphate which is formed resumes a ring structure:

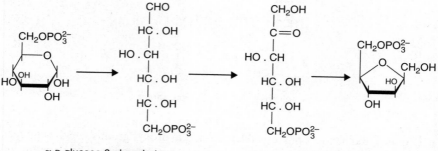

α-D-glucose 6-phosphate   α-D-fructose 6-phosphate

Appendix 2
Enzyme kinetics and the regulation of reactions

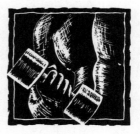

Enzymes speed up the rate of specific chemical reactions, allowing them to be regulated in a way that permits the body to control the interactions between the different metabolic pathways that sustain life. The direction in which the reactions proceed and the equilibrium point that would be reached in a non-biological system are governed by the laws of thermodynamics. The most striking feature of enzyme-catalysed reactions is that they can reach the point of saturation: at low concentrations of substrate, the initial reaction rate increases linearly in response to increasing substrate concentration, but the rate approaches a limit above which it is constant and independent of substrate concentration (Fig. A2.1). The characteristics of enzymes that cause this behaviour are described briefly here.

A2.1 Mechanisms of enzyme action

Thermodynamics tells us that chemical reactions proceed spontaneously only in the direction that results in the products of the reaction having a lower energy

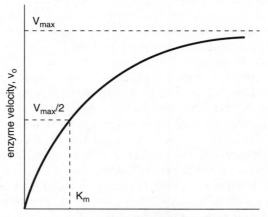

Fig. A2.1 The effect of substrate concentration on enzyme activity.

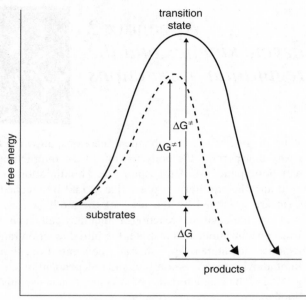

Fig. A2.2 The total free energy of the reaction products is less (by an amount equal to ΔG) than that of the substrates. In order to allow the reaction to proceed, however, sufficient energy to overcome the Energy Activation ($\Delta G°$) is available.

status than the substrates (Fig. A2.2). Enzymes function by acting as re-usable catalysts: this involves the formation of an enzyme–substrate complex as an intermediate step in the reaction. The formation of this intermediate step lowers the energy of activation. Because less energy now has to be added, the reaction is more likely to proceed. It is important to appreciate that the enzyme, although it participates in the reaction, is not consumed and is, therefore, required to be present in only small amounts.

The energetics of the formation of the enzyme–substrate complex are not well understood, but there is clearly some type of weak bond formed between the substrate and the enzyme. This involves one or more active sites on the enzyme, and these sites have a particular shape and charge distribution that allows them to interact with the substrate. These characteristics allow enzymes to promote the rates of specific reaction in a number of different ways. Where two or more substrates are involved, attachment to binding sites on the enzyme allows the substrates to be brought into close proximity in the correct orientation, thus increasing the chances of a reaction taking place. Alternatively, binding to the enzyme can cause changes in the shape of the substrate molecule that increase its susceptibility to reaction.

A2.2 Enzyme kinetics

The first stage in an enzyme-catalysed reaction is the binding of the substrate (S) to the active site of the enzyme (E) to form an enzyme–substrate complex (ES): the substrate then reacts to form the product (P), which is released. Release of the product restores the enzyme to its original free form. This sequence of reactions can be described as follows:

$$E + S \leftrightarrow ES \rightarrow E + P. \tag{A2.1}$$

The assumption made here is that the first stage of the process is reversible, but that the second is not. In almost all reactions, the concentration of the substrate is far in excess of the enzyme concentration. This means that formation of the ES complex does not result in an appreciable change in the substrate concentration, but it does reduce the concentration of the free enzyme. Each of the reactions will proceed at a rate that is defined by the product of the substrate concentration and the rate constant (k) for that reaction. Thus, the reaction:

$$E + S \rightarrow ES \tag{A2.2}$$

will proceed at a rate that depends on the concentrations of E and S, such that the reaction rate, the rate of change of the substrate concentration with respect to time (t) is described as follows:

$$d[ES]/dt = k[E][S]. \tag{A2.3}$$

When the concentration of the reactants is unity (taken to be 1 mol^{-1}), the rate of the reaction is equal to the rate constant (k).

The rate of formation of the ES complex (eqn A2.3) is thus determined by the rate constant (k_1) and the concentrations of substrate and free enzyme. The rate of the reverse reaction depends on the rate constant (k_2) for that reaction and on [ES]. The rate of dissociation of the ES complex to release the free enzyme and the product (k_3) is also dependent on [ES]:

$$[E] + [S] \underset{k_2}{\overset{k_1}{\rightleftarrows}} [ES] \overset{k_3}{\rightarrow} [E] + [P]. \tag{A2.4}$$

The concentration of free enzyme ([E]) at any time is equal to the total enzyme concentration ([E_o]) minus the concentration of the ES complex. If this reaction is in steady state, the rate of ES formation must be equal to the rate of breakdown, i.e. $k_2[ES]$ is equal to $k_3[ES]$, and it must also follow that the rate of formation of ES, i.e. $k_1[E_{free}][S]$, is equal to the sum of $k_2[ES]$ and $k_3[ES]$:

$$k_1[E][S] = k_2[ES] + k_3[ES]$$
$$= (k_2 + k_3)[ES]. \tag{A2.5}$$

The overall reaction rate (v) is given by:

$$v = k_3 [ES].\tag{A2.6}$$

On rearrangement:

$$[ES] = v/k_3.\tag{A2.7}$$

The highest possible reaction rate (V_{max}) is achieved when the enzyme is completely saturated with substrate, i.e. when $[ES] = [E_o]$, and is equal to $k_3[E_o]$, so that:

$$[E_o] = V_{max}/k_3.\tag{A2.8}$$

Eqn A2.5 can be expressed as follows:

$$k_1 ([E_o] - [ES]) [S] = (k_2 + k_3)[ES].\tag{A2.9}$$

If eqn A2.7 and A2.8 are now substituted in eqn A2.9, we now have:

$$k_1 [S] \cdot (V_{max} - v)/k_3 = (k_2 + k_3) \cdot v/k_3.\tag{A2.10}$$

If both sides of the equation are now multiplied by k_3/k_1;

$$[S] (V_{max} - v) = ((k_2 + k_3)/k_1 + [S]) v.\tag{A2.11}$$

The term $((k_2 + k_3)/k_1)$ in eqn A2.11 is the Michaelis constant (K_m). If both sides of of eqn A2.11 are divided by ($K_m + [S]$), we now have:

$$v = V_{max}[S]/(K_m + [S]).\tag{A2.12}$$

The reaction rate (v) is therefore determined by the maximum reaction rate (V_{max}) which is a function of the enzyme concentration, the substrate concentration ($[S]$), and the Michaelis constant.

As the reaction proceeds, the substrate concentration falls, and the reaction rate decreases. The reaction rate (v) therefore applies only to the initial rate when the substrate concentration remains high and the rate of the backward reaction from P to S is negligible.

It also follows from eqn A2.12 that when the substrate concentration is equal to K_m, the reaction rate will be equal to half of the V_{max}. The K_m value is, therefore, equal to the substrate concentration that will result in the reaction proceeding at one half of the maximum rate. A high K_m value is therefore an indication of low affinity of the enzyme for its substrate: a high substrate concentration is necessary to achieve a reaction rate equal to half of the maximum rate.

High reaction rates will only be achieved when the substrate concentration is relatively high. If [S] is equal to 10 times the K_m, substituting these values into eqn A2.12 tells us that the reaction rate will be 91% of V_{max}, while 99% of the maximum rate will only be achieved when the substrate concentration is 100 times the K_m.

A2.2.1 Zero-, first-, and second-order reactions

The order of a reaction is an expression of the power to which the reactant concentrations are raised in the rate equation: where more than one reactant is involved, these powers are added. A reaction that follows zero-order kinetics is thus essentially independent of substrate concentration. A first-order reaction is linear with respect to increasing substrate concentration, and the relationship between reaction rate and substrate concentration in a second-order reaction is described by a hyperbola.

A2.3 Enzyme activity

The activity of enzymes can be assessed by the rate of substrate utilization or product formation under standardized conditions. The most common unit of measurement is the International Unit (U or IU). This is the amount of enzyme that will convert 1 μmol of substrate to product in 1 min under the conditions specified for that reaction. Although this is the generally used measure among physiologists, the appropriate SI unit should be used. This is the katal (kat) which is defined as the amount of enzyme that will convert 1 mol of substrate to product in 1 s under optimum conditions. At least part of the reason for the persistence of the IU is the difficulty in defining optimum conditions for the activity of individual enzymes.

A2.3.1 Factors influencing enzyme activity

Enzyme activity is particularly sensitive to temperature, and will increase as the temperature increases. At high temperatures, however, the activity falls sharply and irreversibly because of structural changes caused by denaturation of the protein. Any expression of enzyme activities must, therefore, specify the temperature at which measurements are made: temperatures of 25 ° and 37 °C are normally used as standards. Except in extreme cases of heat illness, body temperature seldom exceeds 41 °C, but this is close to the level at which some enzymes and other proteins are affected.

Changes in the ionization state of an enzyme will affect its affinity for its substrate because of changes in structure or charge distribution at the active site.

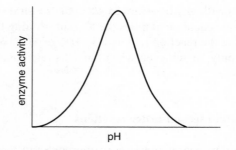

Fig. A2.3 All enzyme regulated reactions are influenced by pH, but the magnitude of the effect and the optimum pH vary widely.

The local pH may also affect the ionization state of the substrate. All enzymes have an optimum pH (Fig. A2.3), but this differs between different enzymes, and may also be influenced by the presence of other activators and inhibitors. Variations in pH are generally small in most tissues, with skeletal muscle showing the largest changes in response to very high-intensity exercise: pH may fall from the resting value of about 7.1 to 6.5 or even less. Many enzymes normally function in an environment that is close to their pH optimum; for example pepsin, which has a pH optimum of about 2.0, seems well adapted for the acid conditions of the stomach. Some enzymes, however, have a pH optimum, at least in their isolated and purified form, that is far from their normal environment; glycerol kinase demonstrates maximum activity at a pH of 9.8, a condition that is never reached in the cell.

A2.3.2 Coenzymes, prosthetic groups, co-factors, and activators

Many enzymes require the presence of one or more coenzymes if the reaction is to proceed: these are compounds which participate in the reaction. The conversion of lactate to pyruvate by lactate dehydrogenase, for example, requires that NAD^+ be available to participate in the reaction. Coenzymes are chemically altered by participation in the reaction, in this case by conversion of NAD^+ to NADH. The coenzyme is, therefore, essentially a substrate for or product of the reaction, but a characteristic of coenzymes is that they are readily regenerated by other reactions within the cell. Some coenzymes, such as NAD^+ are loosely bound to the enzyme, but others (e.g. biotin) are tightly bound and are referred to as prosthetic groups.

Many enzymes have only low activities in the absence of co-factors, and the presence of one or other metal ion, especially the divalent metals calcium, magnesium, manganese, and zinc, is essential for the activation of many enzymes. Binding of these ions alters the charge distribution and shape of the active site of the enzyme. The release of calcium into the cytoplasm in response to the nerve impulse is important in the activation of phosphorylase, which allows acceleration of the glycolytic pathway.

A2.3.3 Competitive and non-competitive inhibition

Substances which have chemical structure similar to that of an enzyme's normal substrate may also be able to bind to the active site on this enzyme and thus interfere with enzyme function by reducing the number of active sites available to the proper substrate. These substances compete with the substrate for access to the active site and are, therefore, referred to as competitive inhibitors. The effect of competitive inhibition is to increase K_m. Increasing the concentration of substrate to a sufficient level will, however, swamp the effects of the inhibitor, and V_{max} is not affected by competitive inhibition.

Non-competitive inhibitors bind to the enzyme at other sites, leaving the active site of the enzyme available to the substrate, but they have the effect of altering the conformation of the protein and thus reducing the catalytic activity of the active site. The V_{max} is reduced, but the same substrate concentration will still produce one half of the new maximum activity, i.e. K_m remains unchanged.

A2.3.4 Allosteric and covalent modulation

Allosteric modulation of enzyme activity refers to the reversible binding of small molecules to the enzyme at sites other than the active site, producing a conformational change in the structure of the enzyme molecule. This change in shape and charge distribution results in a change (either an increase or a decrease) in the affinity of the enzyme for its substrates or products and hence in its activity. Covalent modulation involves phosphorylation or dephosphorylation of an enzyme—usually involving the –OH group of a serine residue in the polypeptide chain. The importance of covalent modulation in controlling the activity of some of the key enzymes of glycolysis is described in Chapter 3.

A2.3.5 Enzyme isoforms

Many enzymes exist in more than one form: these isoforms catalyse the same reaction, but are generally found in different tissues and may have different specificities or catalytic capabilities.

Lactate dehydrogenase exists in two forms, each made up of four subunits. The subunits exist in one of two forms; the H form is found predominantly in cardiac muscle, whereas the M form predominates in skeletal muscle. Five possible different combinations of these subunits are possible. In muscle, the H form is associated with tissues having a high capacity for oxidative metabolism,

Biochemistry of Exercise and Training

and which, therefore, have a high capacity for lactate oxidation, whereas the M form is associated with tissues having a high-anaerobic capacity relative to their oxidative capability. Many other enzymes also exist in a variety of different iso-forms, but the functional significance of these is not well understood.

References

Cornish-Bowden, A. and Wharton, C. W. (1988). *Enzyme kinetics*. IRL Press Oxford.
Ottaway, J. H. (1988). *Regulation of enzyme activity*. IRL Press, Oxford.

Appendix 3
Chemical buffers and control of the acid–base balance

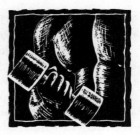

A3.1 Definitions

An acid is a compound able to donate a hydrogen ion (H^+), e.g. HCl, H_2CO_3.
A base is a compound able to accept a hydrogen ion, e.g. HCO_3^-.
pH is the negative decimal logarithm of the free $[H^+]$ concentration (i.e. the concentration of free $[H^+]$ increases 10-fold for each unit decrease of pH).

A fuller working of the steps in the calculation of pH from a known hydrogen ion concentration might aid understanding. The following worked example demonstrates the calculation of the pH of a solution containing 40 nmoles l^{-1} H^+.

$pH = -\log_{10}[H^+]$.

Since $[H^+] = 40$ nmol $l^{-1} = 40 \times 10^{-9}$ mol $l^{-1} = 4 \times 10^{-8}$ mol l^{-1},

$pH = -\log (4 \times 10^{-8})$,
$\log 4 = 0.60$,

so:

$pH = -\log (10^{0.60} \times 10^{-8})$,
$= -\log 10^{-7.4}$,
$= -(-7.4)$,
$= 7.4$.

A3.2 Background

Despite the production of large amounts of carbon dioxide (which leads to the generation of H^+ ions on reaction with water) and of non-volatile acids (as a consequence of metabolism of the nitrogen, sulfur, and phosphorus content of protein) by the body, the extracellular fluid (ECF) is kept slightly alkaline, at a pH of 7.36–7.44. Organic and inorganic constituents of extracellular and intracellular fluids buffer some of the H^+ ions, and the excretion of CO_2 by the lungs and of H^+ by the kidneys disposes of the remainder. These same mechanisms also minimize the change in the pH of the ECF when extra acid or alkali is added.

The processes of buffering and excretion of H^+ ions differ not only in the mechanisms involved, but also in the rate at which they occur. Thus, buffering is a passive, physicochemical process involving near-instantaneous changes in the equilibrium between H^+ ions, the base that binds H^+ and the H^+-base complex (an acid). It limits (or buffers) changes in free H^+ concentration (pH) through changes in bound H^+. However, it cannot prevent some change in pH occurring and it does not affect the total change in H^+ content of the body which occurs when acid or base is added. Excretion of CO_2 or H^+, on the other hand, is a physiological process which responds more slowly than buffering, but in the long term works to restore the total H^+ content of the body to normal after an acid–base disturbance.

The nature and speed of the buffering process means that it is continually changing in response to fluctuations in H^+ load, limiting pH shifts not only immediately after an acid–base disturbance, but also during the period when the physiological response is working to restore a normal body total H^+ content.

A3.3 Buffers

There are both extracellular and intracellular buffers. The principal extracellular buffers are bicarbonate, plasma proteins, and phosphate, and the total amount of buffer available in blood for combination with H^+ is called the buffer base. The intracellular buffers include bicarbonate, proteins, and phosphoric esters. The importance of the intracellular buffers, which are present in all cells, can be illustrated in respect of erythrocytes as follows: when 10 mmol of H^+ are added to a litre of plasma the pH falls from 7.4 to 5.6, but when the same amount of H^+ is added to a litre of blood the pH falls only from 7.4 to 7.0.

For each buffer, the Law of Mass Action states that there will be an equilibrium of the form:

$$[H^+] \cdot [B^-] = K_a \cdot [BH] ; \tag{A3.1}$$

$[B^-]$, $[H^+]$, and $[BH]$ are the concentrations of buffer base, H^+, and acid, respectively. K_a is the dissociation constant of the acid, i.e. the concentration of H^+ at which the concentrations of B^- and BH are equal.

This equilibrium can be re-arranged in the form called the Henderson equation:

$$[H^+] = K_a \cdot [BH] / [B^-]; \tag{A3.2}$$

which describes how the free H^+ concentration depends on the concentrations of base ($[B^-]$) and acid ($[BH]$) present. An alternative form of this equation which is used is that derived by Henderson and Hasselbalch:

$$pH = pK_a + \log_{10}[B^-] / [BH]; \tag{A3.3}$$

where pK_a is the negative logarithm to the base 10 of K_a, i.e. the pH at which the concentrations of acid ([BH]) and base ([B$^-$]) are equal.

When this equation is applied to the bicarbonate–carbonic acid buffer system, a modified form is used. Since carbonic acid is also in equilibrium with water and CO_2, the concentration of carbonic acid present depends directly on the concentration of dissolved CO_2 and on the equilibrium constant of this reaction. As a result, the Henderson–Hasselbalch equation for the bicarbonate–carbonic acid system can be rewritten as:

$$pH = 6.1 + \log [HCO_3^-]/(S \cdot CO_2). \tag{A3.4}$$

In this equation S is the solubility of CO_2 in water (1 kPa partial pressure produces a concentration of dissolved CO_2 of 0.226 mmol^{-1} at 37 °C) and the value 6.1 allows for the dissociation constant of the reaction between carbonic acid and CO_2 + water.

Approximate average values in healthy persons are:

$$7.4 = 6.1 + \log 24/(0.226 \times 5.3). \tag{A3.5}$$

It is sometimes easier to use [H$^+$] directly rather than pH in which case the relationship is the other way up (given by the Henderson equation, see above):

$$[H^+] = k \cdot pCO_2 /[HCO_3^-]. \tag{A3.6}$$

Normal values for [H$^+$], pCO_2, and [HCO$_3^-$] are 40 nM, 5.3 kPa (40 mmHg), and 24 mmol^{-1}, respectively, so that normally:

$$40 = k \cdot 5.3/24; \tag{A3.7}$$

which gives k equal to 181.1.

From this it follows that when the buffer system is at equilibrium, which occurs very rapidly (within a few seconds), the pH depends on the ratio of HCO$_3^-$ to pCO_2 (which will be called the bicarbonate/CO$_2$ ratio from now on). Thus, a rise in HCO$_3^-$ or a fall in pCO_2, which both increase this ratio, cause an increase in pH (i.e. more alkaline conditions) while a fall in HCO$_3^-$ or a rise in pCO_2 decrease pH (i.e. more acid conditions). For example, if pCO_2 were increased to 6 kPa, [H$^+$] would be given by:

$$[H^+] = 181.1 \cdot (6.0/24) = 45 \text{ nM}. \tag{A3.8}$$

Thus, an increase in pCO_2 leads to an increase in [H$^+$]. For many purposes the size of the change does not need to be calculated and it is sufficient just to determine the direction of the change in [H$^+$] caused by particular shifts in pCO_2 or [HCO$_3^-$] from normal. In this case, a simplified form of the relationship can be used:

$$[H^+] \propto pCO_2/[HCO_3^-]. \tag{A3.9}$$

From this relationship it can be seen that a rise in [H$^+$] could result from an increase in pCO$_2$ or a decrease in [HCO$_3^-$] or both, etc.

The bicarbonate–carbonic acid buffer system is the most important in the body. This seems strange at first sight since a buffer system is generally considered to work best in the range ±1 pH unit from the pK$_a$. Thus, with an overall pK$_a$ of 6.1, the normal blood pH (about 7.4) is outside the optimal buffering range for this system. Two features of the system make it so important:

1. There is a large amount of it so that reasonably large changes in the amount of H$^+$ bound can still occur when H$^+$ ions are added or removed,
2. The system is open so that the amounts of the components of the buffer system are not constant, but can change with the needs of the body.

Of these two features, the second is the more important. The significance of the open system can be seen most easily by comparing the properties of closed and open systems. In a closed system, none of the components can exchange with the surroundings, i.e. as if it were contained in a sealed vessel. The total amount of B is, therefore, fixed so that the sum of acid + base (i.e. [BH] + [B$^-$]) is constant. If H$^+$ is added to the system, H$^+$ will rapidly combine with B$^-$ to form BH so that [BH] rapidly increases and [B$^-$] decreases. This process continues until the accumulation of [BH] and depletion of [B$^-$], which tend to drive the reaction in the reverse direction, are sufficient to counteract this process. A new equilibrium state is, therefore, rapidly established in which no further buffering of H$^+$ (i.e. combination with a base) occurs and this will determine the final pH in the system.

In an open system one (or more) of the components can exchange with the surroundings so that its concentration can vary independently of that of other components. The ECF bicarbonate-buffer system in the body is open since CO$_2$, H$^+$, and HCO$_3^-$ can all exchange with the surroundings. Carbon enters the body in the form of food, which is metabolized to CO$_2$ by cells, and is excreted by the lungs. H$^+$ enters both as acids in the diet and as products of metabolism and is excreted by the kidneys. HCO$_3^-$ is created in cells from CO$_2$ and H$_2$O in the presence of carbonic anhydrase and can be lost or generated by the kidneys. The accumulations and depletions of B$^-$ and BH which occur in the closed system on addition (or removal) of H$^+$ can, therefore, be prevented by movement of B or BH (or H$^+$ itself) into or out of the system. This maintains conditions in which buffering of H$^+$ can continue.

In the body, entry of CO$_2$ and H$^+$ in the diet cannot be avoided and the acid–base balance is, therefore, regulated primarily via the excretory processes. These can be varied largely independently of each other through physiological control mechanisms, with the result that both numerator and denominator of the Henderson equation can be altered. This provides physiological control of ECF pH. In the short term, regulation of CO$_2$ excretion is more important than changes in H$^+$ excretion or modification of HCO$_3^-$ concentration because of its speed and size. The respiratory system usually responds much faster than the kidneys and can excrete an extra 40 mmoles of CO_2 per min compared with about 0.15 mmoles H^+ per min by the kidneys. (Note, however, that the location of the principal chemoreceptor beyond the 'blood–brain barrier' means that the onset of and recovery from some disturbances can be delayed by ionic differences between the blood and CSF.) The kidneys' ability to vary H^+ and bicarbonate handling is vital both to restore a normal ECF HCO_3^- concentration in the long term and to provide acid–base regulation when the disturbance is respiratory in origin, i.e. when hypoventilation causes CO_2 retention.

3.4 Responses to disturbances of the acid–base balance

It is simplest, at least initially, to think of the response to a disturbance of the acid–base balance in two parts. The first is a rapid change in H^+ buffering which absorbs much of the alteration in total H^+ concentration and minimizes the change in free H^+ concentration. This primary response is followed by the slower physiological responses, a change in CO_2 excretion by the lungs (respiratory response) and a change in H^+ and HCO_3^- handling by the kidneys (renal response). To see the effects of these processes, consider first the reactions to a simple disturbance, namely the addition of acid to the ECF (a disturbance similar to that occurring in diabetes mellitus).

3.4.1 Buffering (primary) response

The addition of acid is equivalent to adding H^+ to the left-hand side of the reaction:

$$H^+ + HCO_3^- \rightarrow H_2CO_3 \rightarrow H_2O + CO_2$$
$$+$$
$$B^-$$
$$\downarrow$$
$$BH;$$

where B^- represents the other buffer systems besides HCO_3^-. Some of the added H^+ will bind to HCO_3^- to form carbonic acid and some of this, in turn, will form CO_2 and water. Some H^+ will also be buffered by binding to B^- to form BH. In a closed system, a new equilibrium would be attained with a lower HCO_3^- concentration and a raised pCO_2 and from the equations in the previous section, this change in the bicarbonate/CO_2 ratio would correspond to a fall in pH (by the Henderson–Hasselbalch version of the equation) or a rise in free H^+ concentration (from the Henderson equation). Thus, in spite of the buffers, not all the added H^+ would have become bound so that there is still an increase in the concentration of free H^+ ions in the system.

3.4.2 Physiological (secondary) responses

(i) Respiratory excretion of CO_2

The decrease in pH and increase in alveolar and arterial pCO_2 produce a rapid stimulation of ventilation which exports some CO_2 from the system and so reduces pCO_2. This loss of CO_2 can occur because the system we are dealing with is open. The result is an increase in the bicarbonate/CO_2 ratio which raises the pH from what is was immediately after acid addition and buffering and returns it towards its normal value. Thus, in this case the appropriate respiratory response is a fall in pCO_2 and this would be called a *respiratory compensation* for the disturbance.

(ii) Renal excretion of H^+ (reabsorption of HCO_3^-)

In the same way that respiration can modify the bicarbonate/CO_2 ratio by changing ECF CO_2 concentration in the open buffer system, so the kidney can modify the ratio by altering the bicarbonate concentration. This is a consequence of the primary action of the kidney to secrete H^+ ions. These H^+ ions meet three fates. Many react with bicarbonate in the tubular fluid to form carbonic acid and thence CO_2 and water. These enter the tubular cell where they re-form to H^+ and HCO_3^-. The H^+ is then available for re-secretion and the HCO_3^- enters the blood. By this means, most of the filtered HCO_3^- is 'effectively' reabsorbed under normal conditions. Note that this process does not constitute H^+ excretion since it all takes place within the kidney and the H^+ involved in this cycle does not leave the body.

Of the rest of the H^+ secreted, some is excreted as free H^+ ions (urine pH may fall as low as 4.8), but most is excreted in combination with bases (i.e. buffered). The most important of these reactions in urine are:

$$HPO_4^{2-} + H^+ \rightarrow H_2PO_4^-,$$
and
$$NH_3 + H^+ \rightarrow NH_4^+.$$

NH_3 in the second reaction arises largely from the renal deamination of glutamine.

(*Note regarding the role of carbonic anhydrase*: this enzyme is present in the cytoplasm of tubular cells and, in the proximal tubule, on the luminal surface of the brush border of the cells. It catalyses the conversion of water + CO_2 to carbonic acid and vice versa. Without this enzyme, this reaction occurs relatively slowly and limits the rates at which both the H^+ secretion and HCO_3^- reabsorption can occur.)

When ECF pH is low, as in the present example, H^+ secretion by the kidney is stimulated. This is consistent with the body's need to lose the excess $[H^+]$ and results in the reabsorption of any bicarbonate still remaining in the tubular fluid and an increased excretion of H^+, either as free H^+ ions or bound to urinary buffers. An additional consequence of this increased H⁺ loss in the urine is the generation of 'new' bicarbonate and to see how this happens, we must look again at the mechanism of H⁺ secretion.

Since the H⁺ ions secreted by the renal tubular cells are generated in the cells from the dissociation of carbonic acid, their production is accompanied by the production of a stoichiometrically equivalent amount of HCO_3^- ions. These pass into the blood regardless of the fate of the secreted H⁺ ion. If the secreted H⁺ ion binds to a HCO_3^- ion in the tubular fluid and the resulting molecules of water + CO_2 are reabsorbed, then the overall process is equivalent to reabsorption of the bicarbonate ion from the filtered fluid. However, ions secreted into tubular fluid, from which all the bicarbonate has already been reabsorbed, are excreted in the urine as free H⁺ ions or bound to buffers. In these cases, the movement of bicarbonate from tubular cell to blood, which occurs during H⁺ secretion, is not accompanied by removal of bicarbonate from the tubular fluid and is, therefore, equivalent to the addition of 'new' bicarbonate to the blood. By this mechanism, the kidneys are effectively restoring bicarbonate previously lost in buffering the H⁺ load of the disturbance.

Thus, in summary, the appropriate renal response (called the *renal compensation*) to an acid load is an increased secretion of H⁺, resulting in the increased excretion of free and bound H⁺ and the generation of HCO_3^- in the ECF. The latter increases ECF HCO_3^- concentration and hence the bicarbonate/CO_2 ratio. This, in turn, lowers the H⁺ concentration as predicted by the Henderson equation. (*Note*: the anion of the added acid, e.g. Cl⁻ or SO_4^{2-}, is also excreted in the urine. This occurs more rapidly than the increase in H⁺ excretion and occurs at first with Na⁺ or K⁺ rather than with H⁺.)

Now consider a different acid–base disturbance, a rise in ECF pCO_2. Increased pCO_2 drives the following reaction to the right causing the formation of [H⁺] and bicarbonate:

$$CO_2 + H_2O \rightarrow H_2CO_3 \rightarrow H^+ + HCO_3^-$$
$$+$$
$$B^-$$
$$\downarrow$$
$$BH$$

The primary response in this situation is that other buffer systems rapidly bind some of this H⁺ thus minimizing the pH change which occurs and producing a new equilibrium where there is still a somewhat raised pCO_2, an increased H⁺ concentration, and increased concentrations of HCO_3^- and BH. The binding of H⁺ to B⁻ actually tends to increase the amount of HCO_3^- formed since it mops up H⁺ and so increases the conversion of H_2CO_3 to H⁺ and HCO_3^-. This will, therefore, increase the bicarbonate/CO_2 ratio and so tend to reduce the fall in pH caused by the disturbance. (Note that there is no change in total buffer base since an HCO_3^- is formed for each B⁻ used up. In addition, since the concentration of HCO_3^- is so much larger than that of $[H^+]$ and of the other buffers, the relative change in HCO_3^- concentration in this type of disturbance is, in the short term, rather small. Therefore, in acute respiratory disturbances, the CO_2 change is the thing to look for.) The new state is once again described by the Henderson (or Henderson–Hasselbalch) equation.

The secondary response in a case like this may be renal only, since it may be impairment of the respiratory system which is responsible for the original disturbance. In the long term, however, the raised pCO_2 and lowered ECF pH lead to the generation of HCO_3^- by the kidney, which gradually increases ECF $[HCO_3^-]$ and so raises ECF pH. If the respiratory system can respond normally, ventilation will be stimulated (by the raised pCO_2 and low pH) and excretion of CO_2 increased, thus reducing pCO_2 and raising both the bicarbonate/CO_2 ratio and the pH before any renal response can become evident.

The mechanisms just described work in a similar but opposite way when pCO_2 is altered by hyperventilation. This causes a fall in pCO_2 in the blood and an increase in blood pH which is less than predicted from the change in pCO_2 because the shift of the balance of the reaction to the left causes a decrease in $[HCO_3^-]$.

3.5 'Normal values' and forms of acid–base disturbance

The values normally reported by clinical laboratories are those for pH and pCO_2 for arterial blood, together with a corresponding computed value for $[HCO_3^-]$. The conventional normal values are:

pH: 7.35 to 7.45;
PCO_2: 4.7 to 6.4 kPa (35–48 mmHg);
$[HCO_3^-]$: 23 to 28 mmol l^{-1}.

A pH below the lower limit of 7.35 (i.e. $[H^+]$ of $10^{-7.35}$ M or 45 nmol^{-1}) is described as *acidaemia*, while one above pH 7.45 (i.e. $[H^+]$ below 35 nM) would be *alkalaemia*. This simply states the existence of a frank disturbance of free $[H^+]$ in the blood, and takes no account of the possibility that small deviations may represent significant changes of whole-body $[H^+]$ which have been substantially offset by buffering and physiological responses. *It is, therefore, important to use the* pCO_2 and $[HCO_3^-]$ to determine both the underlying primary disturbance and the extent of any compensatory response that may accompany it.

Any rise in free H^+ levels, even if prevented by compensation from exceeding the normal limit, would indicate an *acidosis* which means an increase in the total H^+ content of the body; its converse is an *alkalosis*. If the *acidosis* were accompanied by a rise in pCO_2 above the normal level then a *respiratory acidosis* would be present. Any rise in $[HCO_3^-]$ concentration above normal would limit the pH deviation, and would, therefore, suggest a partially *compensated respira-*

tory acidosis. Remember that renal responses are rather slow, so that if there is a compensatory rise in HCO_3^- concentration in what is clearly a respiratory acidosis, the acidosis must have existed for some time.

Similarly, a somewhat low pH accompanied by a low $[HCO_3^-]$, but not a rise in pCO_2, would point to an addition of H^+ directly, i.e. not primarily due to respiratory deficiency. This would be called a *metabolic acidosis*. If it was accompanied by a pCO_2 that was below normal, it would be a *compensated metabolic acidosis*, i.e. reduced by a raised ventilation.

A low pH accompanied by both a subnormal HCO_3^- concentration and a pCO_2 above normal would be described as a *mixed respiratory and metabolic acidosis*.

Acknowledgement

This appendix is a modified extract (with permission) from Nottingham University's Bachelor of Medical Sciences Laboratory Handbook.

Index

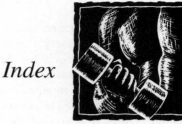